# embody eating

## RECIPES, CHINESE MEDICINE, AND BEYOND

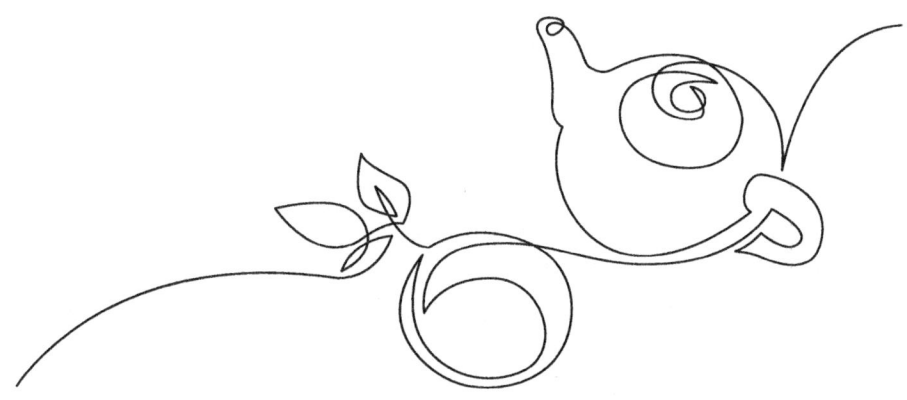

### BETH BRIGHT
MS, L.Ac., Dipl. Ac.

# Endorsements

"First of all, I appreciate Beth Bright as an embodied Buddisatva Goddess energy as well as a healer. Her book made this embodied wisdom accessible and applicable to anyone who is interested in improving their quality of life or developing a muscle for spiritual growth. I highly recommend her book — it can transform your life!"

> – *Master Mingtong Gu, Founder of The Chi Center and The Center for Wisdom Healing Qigong in Santa Fe, NM, USA. Named Qigong Master of the Year by the 13th World Congress for Qigong and Traditional Chinese Medicine.*

"It is a simple but vital question: What should I eat for health? The answer is often confusing or contradictory because of modern information overload and narrow reductionist views. This book allows us to access holistic common sense based on the natural wisdom of Chinese medical principles. We gain practical insight into the how, why, and when of optimal nutrition and mindful digestion — even the philosophy and psychology of food."

> – *Dr. Paul C. Wang, Doctor of Acupuncture and Chinese Medicine, LAc*
> *Instructor of Si Yuan Balance Method*
> *Transmitter of Dao De Gong Fa*
> *Founder of Dao Center*

"Beth Bright has dedicated her professional life to developing practical applications in medicine as an acupuncturist and mind-body health practitioner. Her tireless pursuit to assist others and resolve complicated medical issues leaves no rock unturned. Beth is known to have the courage and humility to look within and turn over a new leaf in life, encouraging others to do the same. She might just have you cook up that leaf for dinner! Read her book to increase the ease of healthy living for you and your family."

> – *Mary White, Heart-Centered Meditation Teacher*

"Attend to this meeting of cultures in the kitchen: It is more than delicious, as food is foundational to health. Beth Bright shares the provender of her Eastern journey, with a gift for making foreign concepts and foods readily accessible."

> – *David Kailin, MPH, PhD Author, Quality in Complementary & Alternative Medicine.*

"Beth Bright has provided me with a 20-year history of confident, caring, intuitive, and successful solutions to my health issues, practicing a comforting Love and Logic approach. This long overdue book will be a helpful treasure to many."

> – *Jim Fay, Author and Co founder, Love and Logic Institute, Inc.*

# table of contents

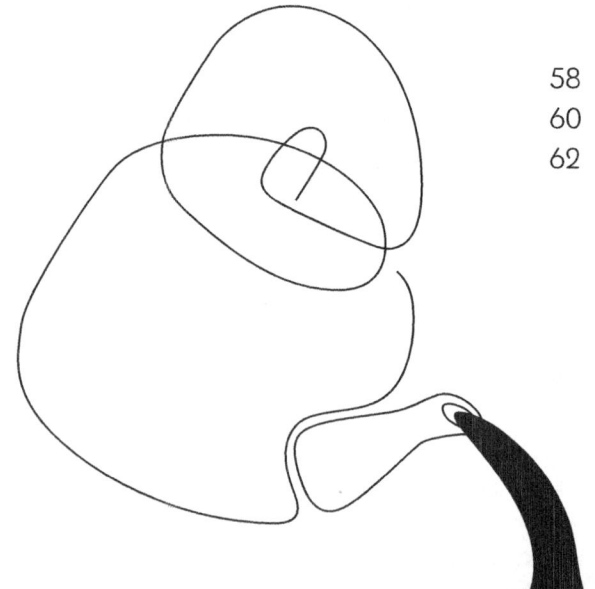

**Ying Recipes cont'd**

**Wei Recipes**

**Appendices**

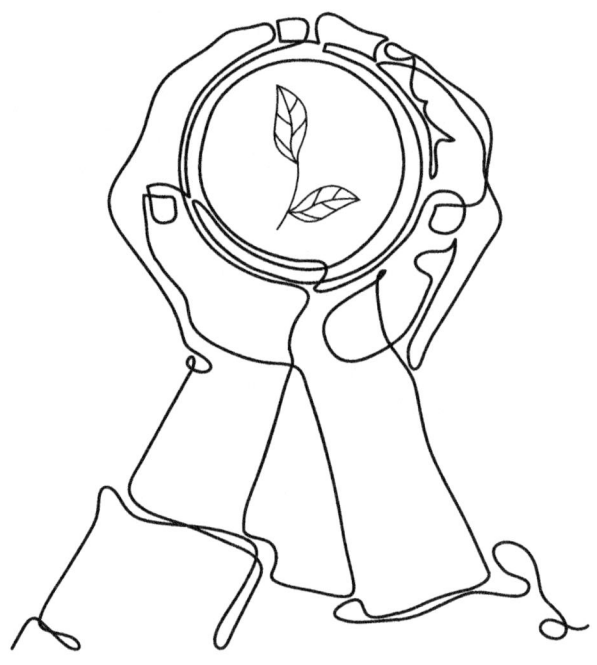

# Friends From Forever

by David Kailin


We are friends from forever
and you have been long away on a far journey.

Now you are home once again
it is morning and the house is very quiet-
everyone else is on vacation-
except the dog, snoozing in a patch of sun.

You serve a bowl of congee
with just one or two herbs added
and a cup of tea with the leaves left in it.

We chat, and you gently explain
the sensibilities of these foods
with wisdom hidden in a bowl of soup
the cultural situation of a glistening spoonful.

We will meet many times just like this
each time over different recipes
with your commentaries gradually guiding and
deepening my experience and understanding.

# Embody Eating: Welcome!

After more than 25 years in clinical practice as a doctor of Chinese Medicine,* the single most common question I am asked is, "What should I eat?".

In Traditional Chinese Medicine (TCM), we look at the collective, energetic influence foods deliver. We think about food entering certain organ pathways in the body and moving in particular directions (inwardly, toward the surface, downwardly, etc.). Foods provide particular qualities such as warming or cooling to the body. Note that I'm not talking about the ambient temperature of the food; I'm talking about the energetics of the foods.

Food is important for good health. We are bombarded with many different diet "cures" for health issues. It is often difficult to sort out all of the options, to figure out what we need, and how to achieve health.

Fortunately, Traditional Chinese Medicine holds a deep understanding of nutrition and food. In fact, our herbal medicine pharmacy is considered to be an extension of food — basically, the "medicine" is actually food that doesn't taste good enough to eat! This ancient health practice offers a thorough knowledge of plant, animal, and mineral life that sustains and heals us. There is also a thorough knowledge of good digestion and how to achieve it. When we eat healthy food and have a healthy digestive system, then we have good nutrition. Nutrition is the result of healthy food and a healthy digestive system nourishing us.

**How to Use This Cookbook**

This is not your average cookbook! You will not find recipes divided by breakfast, lunch, and dinner — or by main dishes, side dishes, and desserts. I have organized this cookbook into three sections: Yuan, Ying, and Wei. These are levels that TCM uses to describe where our food comes from and how it influences the body. Learning which foods belong in each level will help you understand the energetic healing qualities
of your food:

- **Yuan:** Recipes in the Yuan section focus on ingredients that mostly come from the waters.
- **Ying:** Recipes in the Ying section focus on ingredients that come from the land. This is where, by far, the biggest selection of our food comes from. It incorporates the foods we eat the most, so this section has the most recipes.
- **Wei:** Recipes in the Wei section focus on ingredients that mostly come from the sky.

You'll discover more about each level in the following pages.

**Food, Energy, and Medicine**

Each recipe has a section that details some of my understanding of the Traditional Chinese Medicine food energetic system. As you cook the recipes you will gain new appreciation of the energy the food contains. You may even find pleasure in simply handling your food, learning how it is exerting its life force influence on you, and discovering how you feel as a result. Using the various cooking techniques will be fun and you'll learn how to employ them to create the conditions for the health that you want.

And when you eat what you cook, I hope you experience the energy signature of the food, found in the flavors, colors, and growth patterns that make up the food.

I've tried to include recipes that are both easy to shop for and easy to make. I kept families in mind when choosing these recipes, so you can teach your children how to enjoy good food and establish healthy eating habits.

Join me in the garden, kitchen, and at the table as we explore how to experience the energy of food and ourselves. I hope that, together, we may journey into the world of embodied eating and cultivate techniques to grow our health and happiness in life! When we want to change our life, we can begin by changing our food.

This book is dedicated to the highest benefit of healing for you, and all life!

Happy Eating,
Beth Bright, M.S., L.Ac., Dipl.Ac.

*My mentors were mainly Chinese, therefore I refer to what I practice as "Traditional Chinese Medicine." But this is one aspect of what is commonly known as "Traditional East Asian Medicine."*

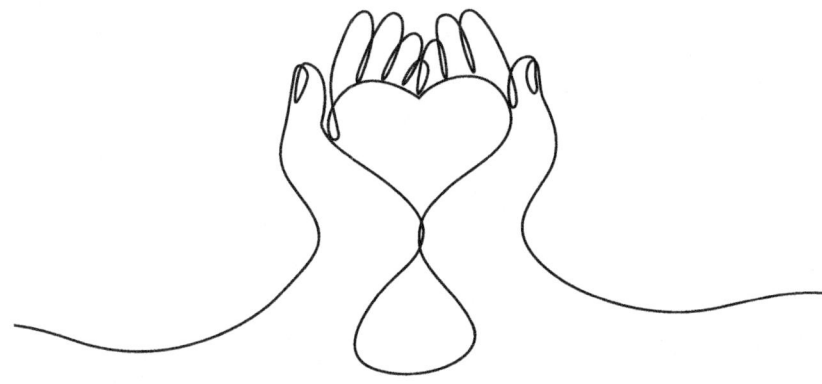

# Embodying Chinese Medicine: Food Energetics, the Yin & Yang of Food, and the Five Elements

Traditional Chinese Medicine provides a unique perspective on food. In this ancient modality, we embrace all food as healthy — as long as it is real food, having lived a life of its own as a plant or an animal. The question is not, "Is this food good or bad?" — rather it is: "What is the relationship between what I'm eating and how I feel?"

## No Bad Foods

Although we don't think of foods as categorically "good" or "bad," we recognize that food is often the cause of disease. This is because some people need foods that they do not eat; or they eat foods that they do not need. The power of TCM lies in its understanding of the energetic functions food provides and how to apply this to what you need in order to enjoy health and vitality!

When you visit a doctor of TCM, you may be given food recommendations to eat as part of your healing regimen. If you are committed to a particular diet — no matter what diet you're following (vegetarian, vegan, or paleo diet, etc.) — they will identify foods that work within that diet to address your health needs.

## Experiential Aspects of Food Energetics

How do we know what is helpful to eat at any time? This is a very interesting question and the beginning of the discovery of experiencing food energetics!

First, let's play with the aspects of warming and cooling...

Have you ever eaten a chocolate bar and felt the heat sensation in your mouth from it? Or had a cup of dark roasted coffee and felt the heat in your mouth, even several minutes after you've swallowed a sip? I'm not talking about the temperature of the coffee, I'm talking about the warming effect it creates in your mouth. Have you ever taken a shot of whiskey and felt the burning sensation in your throat? Even if the whiskey is served cold with ice cubes, it still burns in your throat! How about eating raw garlic or ginger? Even though they may be room temperature, they still burn in your mouth.

Have you ever eaten a handful of lettuce and felt the coolness and moisture in your mouth? What about eating a fresh pear and feeling the cool sensation in your mouth? Have you eaten warm, baked pears and felt their coolness, regardless of their temperature from the oven? Or have you ever chewed on fresh mint or had a cup of mint tea and felt the cold in your mouth?

## Moving away from hot and cold, let's explore flavors...

Have you ever sucked on a lemon and felt your mouth pucker from the sourness? Have you ever eaten dill pickles, or chugged pickle juice, and experienced the sour overload so much that your jaw muscles hurt? What about eating spicy peppers and feeling your face get hot and seeing it turn red? Have you eaten pungent, spicy Thai or Mexican food and felt your sinuses open and your nose clear as you eat your meal?

These experiences of hot, cold, sour, and spicy delivered by the flavors are living examples of "yin" and "yang."

### What are Yin & Yang?
Foods that are heating to your mouth and body are classified as "yang" foods. Foods that are cooling to your mouth and body are classified as "yin" foods.

### But what does that mean?
Yin and yang describe relative opposites, they are a duality. They are mutually dependent and they both create and destroy each other. Typically, "yin" energy is associated with qualities of coolness, moistness, stillness, inward and downward movement, darkness. Typically, "yang" energies have the qualities of heat, dryness, activity, upward and outward movement, lightness.

### Yin & Yang in the Experience of Food
Flavors of food have an energetic quality of yin or yang, too. The sour taste of the lemon and the experience of drawing inwardly with a pucker is an example of the contraction of energy. If you eat enough of anything sour (like that pickle juice) your jaw muscles will contract and hurt! This is an astringent quality of the food, associated with yin energy moving inward.

On the other hand, the spicy, pungent flavor of Thai or Mexican food moves our energy upward to the nose and face, and outward to the skin, turning it red. If you are not used to it, this sensation can be very strong and uncomfortable! It is an example of the "dispersing" quality of yang, moving energy up and out to the surface.

If you eat too much hot, spicy food and feel heat in your stomach, you are eating in a way that creates an "imbalance" of too much yang heat. To soothe and cool the heat, you might eat some watermelon slices, which are a cooling, yin food. This would restore balance and harmony to your stomach.

### Yin & Yang In the Body
In a healthy body, there is a balance and flow between yin and yang. One measure of good health is balance in all body systems — with no single system needing more care than any other system. Chinese Medicine values "balance" and "harmony" in our body organs, body systems, emotions, and in nature and the world. We see everything in terms of relationships. The Universe and Humans are One" - this is a primary concept in Chinese philosophy that means that humans are a part of the larger Universe and nature, and all life is deeply interconnected.

### What are the Five Elements?
There is another classification system for food in TCM called the Five Element System. The five elements are fire, earth, metal, water, and wood.

Each of the five elements has its own quality of energy or qi (pronounced "chee" and sometimes spelled as "chi"). Through careful observation and experience of nature, the TCM perspective classifies food as belonging to one or more of these elements.

It doesn't stop there, the Five Elements is also used to classify body organs, colors, directions, odors, and sounds. It is also used to define how the elements are interconnected and how they influence each other as their own elemental "chemistries" combine. But for this book, we'll focus on how the elements apply to our food and what that means for cooking and healing!

# The organs, colors, qualities, and seasons commonly associated with each of the Five Elements

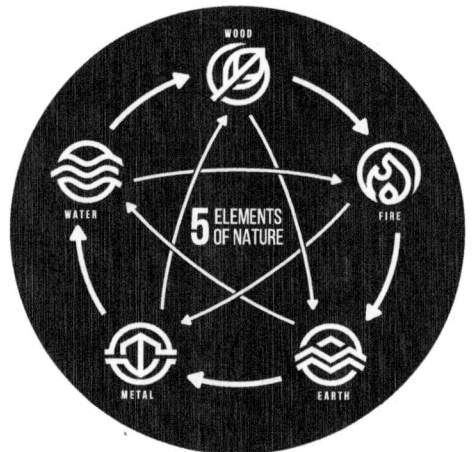

## Water

The water element is associated with:
- The kidneys and urinary tract/bladder
- Salty flavor, purple or dark blue foods
- Foods that grow downward and inwardly
- Nourishing bones and the endocrine system
- Winter

## Wood

The wood element is associated with:
- The liver and gallbladder
- Sour flavor, green-colored food
- Food that grows upwardly
- Nourishing tendons and ligaments
- Spring

## Fire

The fire element is associated with:
- The heart and small intestine
- Bitter flavor, red-colored foods
- Foods that grow up and outwardly
- Nourishing the blood vessels
- Summer

## Metal

The metal element is associated with:
- The lungs and large intestine
- Pungent or spicy flavor, white-colored foods
- Foods that grow downwardly
- Nourishing the skin
- Autumn

## Earth

The earth element is associated with:
- The stomach, pancreas, and spleen
- Sweet flavor, yellow/orange foods
- Food that grows spherically
- Nourishing muscles
- Late summer

Another way to think about the earth is in relation to seasons throughout the yearly calendar.

Earth exerts its influence for a two-week period between each of the four main seasons.

# Yuan, Ying, & Wei

This cookbook is divided into three parts: Yuan, Ying, and Wei. These are three Chinese words that describe three levels of life. Food that grows on these three different levels provides different energies to support our existence. The stomach's job is to transform food — no matter what level the food comes from — so it nourishes the entire body.

## Yuan

*External (environmental):* Yuan describes the deepest and most inward source of energy. It contains the creative, reproductive, essential energy in the environment and in our human bodies. The beginning of all life on planet earth came from the waters, the oceans of life, the "yuan" dimension. As life evolved to breathe air and move onto land, the "ying" dimension evolved.

*Internal (within the body):* Yuan qi is defined as the constitutional energy level, the home of Jing qi that provides the essential energy for life. It includes reproductive energy and the physical substance of this energy in the form of sperm and eggs and their fluids. Jing qi resides at the base of the body. It is the power for supporting life force and vitality. It animates the kidneys, urinary/bladder, reproductive organs, bones and spine. Jing qi is partly acquired from our parents (through DNA), and partly acquired from adequate food, rest, and lifestyle. This also means it is consumed by poor food and lifestyle choices, as well as inadequate rest.

## Ying

*External (environmental):* Ying describes the level of energy that is nourishing and sustaining for life, the middle ground. It is about the foundation of earth as the source of nourishment — the soil, fields of crops, and the animals that sustain all life. This is where most food comes from (and why this is the largest section in this cookbook!)

*Internal (within the body):* The Ying qi level houses nutritive qi. This is the energy that fuels the digestive system and is supported by nutrition. Nutrition is the combination of food and digestion. Thus, nutritive qi is strong when proper food and a healthy digestive system work together. The Ying qi dimension animates the digestive organs: stomach, pancreas, spleen, small intestine, large intestine, and supports the liver and gallbladder. Nutritive qi enables healthy repair of tissues, muscles, tendons, as well as ligaments, blood, and bones. All systems of the body rely on nutritive qi to keep them going.

## Wei

*External (environmental):* Wei describes the upper and outer levels of existence. The outer levels of earth that contain the sky, the higher regions, the tree canopy, and the birds.

*Internal (within the body):* Wei qi is defensive qi. This is the energy of our immune system. Defensive qi protects the body from outside influences that could bring harm, or loss of integrity, to the body's organ and energy systems. Wei qi operates at the most superficial level of the body. It is where the human meets the outer environment. When Wei qi is strong, we are protected from external influences, such as weather, germs, allergens, and parasites. When Wei qi is weak, we are at more risk of being unprotected from outside influences. Wei qi animates the upper body — the head, the heart, the lungs, the respiratory system, the skin, and the sinuses. Wei qi is nourished by proper food (nutritive qi) and rest and exercise (breathing).

# Nutritious Food to Nourish Qi

A healthy diet should accomplish three things. It should nourish energy, support elimination, and promote healing. This means that food needs to give us sustained energy, foods need to strengthen our body. Healthy elimination means one bowel movement per day, in the early morning (5:00-7:00 a.m.), the stool should be formed, easy to produce, and feel complete. "Healing" means that tissue repair and DNA production happens on a continuous, on-going basis.  And, it all begins with good nutrition.

**Good Nutrition & Qi**
Good nutrition is the combination of healthy digestion and proper food. The two revolve around each other. Your digestion needs to be healthy in order to absorb nutrients in foods. Foods need to be nutritious in order to energize your digestion process.

So, what makes food nutritious? According to Traditional Chinese Medicine, food is "nutritious" when it is full of qi. In terms of food, qi is the life force that makes everything, literally every single thing on the planet and in the Universe, form and function and grow. Everything is qi — you are made of qi, nature is made of qi, the Universe is qi. Scientific research has proven this, TCM applies this — and always has! In the body, qi enables tissues and organs and systems to do their jobs. In nature, it is the force of life that makes plants and animals mature and flourish. Qi is the formless energy that makes up at least 96% of the Universe, according to astrophysics.

We gain energy from food in direct proportion to how much qi the food itself contains. Food that has very recently had a life of its own — meaning it was growing and alive, like a vegetable, fruit or animal — is full of energy. The further from being alive and growing that your food becomes, the less energy it contains.

For example, fresh produce that was harvested within the past several days has the most qi to offer. Food that has been frozen (such as frozen vegetables or fruits) had life, but not as recently, thus, not as much qi. And, food that has been processed (such as junk food — Twinkies, Fruit Loops and Cheetos) and no longer resembles anything that was ever alive, has no qi. It is bereft of life and therefore, cannot give any life energy to you when you eat it.

You may be surprised to discover that food that has been canned is also considered processed (think canned green beans, peaches in syrup, or V8 or pineapple juice that sits on the grocery shelf). Even though it was alive long ago, by this point, it also has no qi.

But, home-canned food that was preserved shortly after being harvested and minimally processed, has about as much qi as frozen food.

### Why does it Matter?

The stomach acquires the energy it needs to digest food from the food itself — whatever is in your belly. When your food is not full of qi, the stomach cannot acquire enough energy to break down the food adequately. It must summon assistance from other organs, which tires the body and leads to other problems.

# How to Eat, Embodied

### How to Eat

As simple as it may sound, mentioning *how* to eat is necessary for good digestive health. There are a few fundamental things to practice when it comes to eating.

**First: Relax.** It's important to sit down to eat. Stomach qi runs from the stomach through the legs. So, if you stand up and eat, your stomach qi moves to your legs. When stomach qi is in your legs, it's working to stand you up rather than in your stomach where it is needed to digest your food. So, take a seat when you eat! Next, make eating a pleasant, sensual experience — think about sight and sound as well as taste. Make your dining place lovely to be in. Set your table with a placemat or tablecloth, silverware, napkins, flowers, candles, and relaxing music. Stressful eating environments, as well as internal stress, both lead to digestive disorders. Worry and fear contract our stomach energy which makes it difficult to receive and digest our food. So relax and deeply enjoy your food! In a word: Gratitude for our food helps us relax! The traditional way of saying grace before eating is really a gratitude practice that can help us to center, appreciate, and relax.

**This leads to number two: Focus on eating when eating.** The stomach energy is also the energy that governs focused concentration. When we are reading, studying, or concentrating, the energy of the stomach supplies the qi to keep the mental focus sustained. If we are eating at the same time as reading or watching TV, the stomach energy is diverted away from digesting food. We are now digesting information, instead of food. This creates physical digestion problems. Pleasant, light conversation while eating actually relaxes the stomach and aids digestion. But stressful business meetings during lunches or dinners are a direct cause of digestive disorders! It is the same with reading or studying while eating. Being fully present while eating, with our attention on our food, good posture, enjoying our meal, relaxing, and sharing a little conversation with others enables good digestion.

**Number three, and very important: CHEW WELL!** Patients come to me with digestive complaints, especially gas, bloating, and abdominal discomfort after eating. Often this is cured by chewing food very well. This means chewing around 30–40 times before swallowing. Better yet, chewing until there is nothing left in the mouth to chew — when the food is completely mashed into liquid in the mouth.

Chewing and swallowing happen with the aid of saliva. The purpose of saliva is to begin breaking down food in the mouth, before we swallow. If food doesn't spend enough time in the mouth getting chewed and mixed with saliva, then a big glob of unbroken down food is swallowed and lands in the stomach — and that is uncomfortable and taxing to digest.

Chewing until food is completely liquid in the mouth also helps us eat the right amount. It is almost impossible to overeat when we take the time to thoroughly chew. Overeating is a dominant cause of digestive problems and it accelerates the aging process! It takes a lot of energy to digest food. If we overtax this process, we consume energy instead of conserving it, and we age ourselves faster.

The stomach gains energy from healthy, nutritious food it directly receives. Please eat only until you're 70% to 80% full! The stomach needs room to breathe after eating, so that qi can circulate in order to digest. You will feel good if you stick with this simple guidance. Digestion involves a complex dance of hormones in your blood that signal when the stomach is "full." This requires about 30 minutes. If you eat to 70% to 80% full and you are chewing very well, tasting your food, and feeling your food when you swallow, your meal will take some time. This should be enough time for your hormones to signal to you that you're full. Then, it is likely you will feel satisfied and maybe not even want dessert!

*NOTE: Chewing well includes not talking while chewing. This prevents choking, aids good digestion, and is much more pleasant for dinner partners! Truly! Please do not talk, sing, or laugh with your mouth full!*

**Fourth: Eat at regular times every day.** The body has a rhythm, organ energies cycle in a regular pattern throughout the 24-hour clock. The stomach loves regular feeding, and it thrives on it. A regular eating schedule allows the blood sugar to stabilize, which results in not having cravings. Cravings are often the result of low blood sugar that happens when we skip a meal, get hungry, and want a quick fix. The stomach reaches its peak of energy between 7:00–9:00 a.m. This is why breakfast is so important. It is better to try to eat a little something at regular meal times even if you are not particularly hungry (especially at breakfast), than to skip a meal or eat at irregular times. Constantly eating (aka "grazing)" fatigues the stomach qi, creating digestive problems. The other timing issue is not to eat too close to bedtime. Sleep is the other part of health that thrives on regularity. Eating late at night or within 2 hours of sleeping can really slow digestion and create health problems.

## Be Conscious as You Eat

As you eat more consciously, gradually your food desires will calm down, and your wants become more simple. You will naturally know what you need to eat. You will truly be able to listen to your body. Do not overthink food! Return to your natural state, inside your "home," inside your body. Feeling grateful for food, relaxing, chewing, digesting, and being a natural human is a big deal. It's easy to understand, but may be difficult to experience or achieve. It requires patient practice, really tuning into yourself while eating — i.e. embodied eating!

# What to Eat

TCM takes into account individual needs, constitutions, and health when recommending what to eat. Specific diets can be an important part of healing, and your Chinese Medicine doctor can help you with this. So at the risk of oversimplifying what to eat, here are a few simple and mostly universal guidelines:

- **Eat real food** — food that was alive and growing.
- **Eat grains that you can see,** not processed grains that are unrecognizable as a living grain.
- **Eat fiber!** Fiber makes you feel satisfied. Fiber foods are grains such as oats, brown and wild rice, all vegetables, such as green vegetables, yellow vegetables, fresh fruits, and nuts, seeds, and beans. (NOTE: Bread, white rice, processed foods, meat, fish, eggs, and dairy do not provide any fiber).
- **Avoid fake foods,** especially processed foods, low-fat foods, artificial sweeteners, and high-fructose corn syrup (HFC). Fat has received a bad reputation that is undeserved, the brain needs high-quality fats in order to function well. Think about what it takes to "reduce fat" in a food — processing!!
- **Do not eat foods you are sensitive or allergic to.**
- **If you eat snacks, choose foods that aid digestion** such as high-fiber and low-sugar foods, i.e., fruits and vegetables.

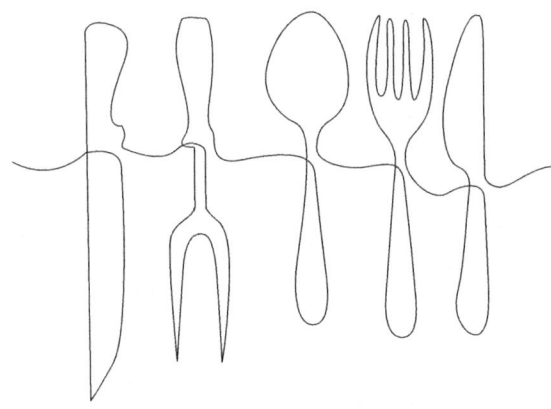

"Feeling grateful for food, relaxing, chewing, digesting, and being a natural human is a big deal."

It is better for the stomach to eat real food that it can recognize thanks to generations of eating. This leads to the concept of "dampness." This is an important and helpful concept in Chinese Medicine.

## What Is Dampness?
Dampness is basically inflammation, swelling (both on the body surface and internally), and fluid stagnation that creates digestion problems, and is a symptom of digestive problems. We may eat and drink things that bring in moisture, but are too difficult to clear out, and so the digestive system gets bogged down and dampness results. The idea is to consume foods that both nourish us, and clean up the digestive tract as we go. Dampness leads to the inability to concentrate, feeling overwhelmed, feeling heavy, lethargic, and gaining weight. How does dampness occur? Mainly from poor eating habits — eating too much sugar (or ANY high-fructose corn syrup), dairy, gluten, fried foods, and alcohol; also eating too much raw, cold food; and overeating or eating when you're not hungry. To clean up dampness, it is recommended to avoid the foods and habits mentioned above, and to cook all food. Be sure to cook and eat green leafy vegetables, green beans, snow peas, mushrooms, sprouts, wild rice, buckwheat, and certain spices such as oregano, cumin, and dill (to name a few) in order to help clear out dampness. You may benefit from adding fermented foods (sauerkraut, kombucha, miso soup, yogurt, etc.) as probiotics to help clear up the digestive tract. Also, do not combine grains or tubers with protein for meals. Dampness occurs as an effort by the stomach to make a substitute for healthy yin fluids. It is good to eat watery foods to solve this issue before it happens! Your TCM doctor will know how to help if dampness is a problem for you.

## A Simple Plan
In general, it is good to follow this simple plan for what to eat (See Meal Suggestions in Appendix pg. 104):
- For breakfast, eat grains and protein.
- For lunch and dinner, eat grains, greens (vegetables), and protein.
- Eat most everything warm/cooked.
- Eat a variety of foods.
- Enjoy fresh fruit by itself as a snack

This means for breakfast, enjoy oatmeal or congee or muesli — (any cooked grain) along with breakfast meat or egg or nuts or occasional yogurt, ie-protein. For lunch and dinner, have any grain with greens — vegetables of all colors really, and more than one vegetable, cooked, and some protein.

## Protein
If you are vegan your protein source will be vegetables, legumes, plus grains, nuts, and seeds. If you are vegetarian your protein source will be legumes (including soy, grains, nuts, seeds) and dairy food. If you are an omnivore, there are many different kinds of protein

sources: meat, fish, bones (bone broths), nuts, seeds, eggs, vegetables (legumes), and dairy. Vegan diets tend to be very cooling, so it is helpful to add warming herbs, spices, and cooking techniques like roasting, barbecuing, or frying, in order to create balance and good digestion. Dairy food is warming and sticky, difficult to digest for many people. So adding green leafy vegetables and warming herbs to move energy is helpful. Eating a little fermented food may also aid digestion of dairy. Meat is warming and can be balanced by eating lots of green vegetables. If you experience noxious smelling gas, you are not digesting protein, especially meat, well.

## Fats

Fats are essential in the diet to nourish hormone production and brain function. Eating high quality fats , such as oily SMASH fish (Sardines, Mackerel, Anchovies, Salmon, Herring) and nuts, seeds, eggs, and beans support kidney yin. If you roast the nuts and seeds, adding heat, they support kidney yang. Both are essential. Balance is the key, depending on what you need.

## Grains

"Grains" means whole grain that you can see, for example rice, not refined grain, like flour. Of course, we substitute "tubers" for grains sometimes - potatoes, sweet potatoes, and yams. This is just fine if the digestive system is strong enough. Helpful (non-glutinous) grains include rice, millet, oats, corn, buckwheat, quinoa, amaranth.

## Fruit

Fruits are an important part of a healthy diet, but in general fruit is hard to digest combined with other foods. So eat fruit as a snack, by itself.

## Variety Is Important

Keep a rotation of many various foods going for meals and snacks and you will gain energy from all three levels — Yuan, Ying, and Wei — and all Five Elements: earth, metal, water, wood, and fire. Cooking methods also contribute to the elements going into the foods. When you rotate what you cook and eat, the digestive tract grows the microbes, or ability, to digest whatever you feed it. A big variety of foods means a big variety of healthy digestive bacteria — and this also strengthens our immune system.

In a way, accepting more variety of foods is a reflection of accepting more variety of life, easily expanding our capacity to enjoy the offerings of Mother Earth. Take in and allow a growing experience of tastes, textures, and flavors without judgment of "good/bad" or "right/wrong" — simply welcome the variety of life that modern-day refrigerated shipping and storage make available. However, eating local produce and foods that are in season is another way to enjoy your food. My point is, when the digestive system is healthy, we are able to eat a variety of foods and enjoy life very much!

*NOTE: After eating a meal that is easy to digest you will feel very comfortable, satisfied, and at ease.*

**One Final Thought**

It is important not to take anything you learn too rigidly. Whatever you may glean from this book, hold it lightly. Do not go to extremes to follow your new knowledge. It boils down to being very simple: eat, sleep, move! This is the basic formula for a healthy life. These are natural states for human beings; do not make them more complicated. While it is true that everyone is different and our acquired needs differ, it is also true that returning to our natural state of "eat, sleep, move" IS being healthy! Enjoy the simplicity and peace of embodied eating for every meal!

# How to Drink, Embodied

Imagine that you are standing at the kitchen counter drinking a cup of hot coffee. You are hungry. It's morning and you've just blended a smoothie for breakfast. You are running late, so you guzzle down half the glass of smoothie while finding your shoes and stressing about the time. You run around looking for your phone, and then take another huge gulp of smoothie, finishing the glass and dashing out the door. You are feeling rushed and your stomach isn't feeling too good.

Now imagine the same scene as if you are inside your stomach. You feel the comfortable body temperature of the stomach organ and the added heat of coffee and stomach acid inside of the stomach. You are noticing tension in the stomach organ from a sense of stressful worry signals. Suddenly, a huge flood of icy, cold, thick smoothie fills your stomach. What a shock! It's like a flash flood of fluid — so cold, so sticky, perhaps sweet too, so uncomfortable! Now you feel your stomach reacting to this shock, there is an urgent demand for more energy in order to warm up the fluid inside your stomach so that it can become digestible. The coldness and stickiness of the smoothie slows down the process of digesting it. The stomach is stressed out and exerting extra energy in order to do its job. And then, GUSH! Another huge flood of cold smoothie hits the stomach, creating more stress and a call for increased energy in order to handle the demand. The stomach qi is contracted from the amount of cold, and unable to flow very well to process the event.

"The stomach wants a steady pace of intake;
   not a rush and gush of floods."

What the stomach really wants from a drink is a gentle, slow sip, followed by another gentle, slow sip. And after finishing a drink (or meal), the stomach needs time to rest for a while, taking in nothing more. The stomach wants fluids that are close to body temperature, so that it doesn't need to exert extra energy to warm up or cool down a fluid in order to be able to digest it. The stomach wants a stream of watery fluids throughout the day, with breaks in between drinking (and eating) when the stomach can rest, and gather qi for meeting its next demand. The stomach wants a steady pace of intake; not a rush and gush of floods. How exhausting!! So slowly drinking, and not guzzling, is ALWAYS appropriate, even if you are very thirsty. Your stomach and entire body will be able to relax and function very well with this simple practice of drinking slowly.

# What to Drink

When it comes to digestion, drinking is as important as eating. Digestion requires a lot of fluid.  How do we get fluids? From eating fresh vegetables and fruits, eating watery cooked foods (such as soups and stews and watery porridges), and from drinking fluids. Let's think about this a little. The body loves water, in fact, water makes up about 60% of our body weight and is 90% of our blood. When we digest water, we absorb water into our blood and organs. It is essential for life. That means that most of our fluid intake needs to be water.

### What about juice?
Juice is popular, and it's watery, right? The problem with drinking juice is that one glass of juice contains more fruit or vegetables than we would ever eat at one time. Juice is very concentrated. Fruit has a very cold effect on the body. If we drink a glass of fruit juice, the stomach is hit with a very large, cold gush of concentrated sweetness. This is extremely hard to digest. It leads to what Chinese Medicine calls "internal dampness," meaning the stomach gets bogged down and cannot function properly. A glass of juice is really a "treatment" similar to an herbal formula being a treatment — because it is so highly concentrated. In general, all fruit has cold energy and does not combine well with other foods. So drinking fruit juice should not occur with eating food in order for the stomach to digest well.

### What happens when we drink milk?
Milk, and dairy food in general, is highly sticky and congesting, it produces phlegm. Milk is also warming in nature. Goat's milk is easier for people to digest than cow's milk.

What we combine with our drinks has a big effect on our stomach. For example, drinking a glass of milk (dairy protein) and eating an orange has a curdling effect. The sticky nature of dairy food combined with the acidity of the orange does not mix well together. They curdle each other and we experience that in our stomach. That means we get stomach pain or nausea from the combination of milk and orange. If we persist in the habit of bad food and drink combinations, over time, it can create more serious conditions such as irritable bowel syndrome (IBS).

### What about adding a protein powder?

Protein powders are popular, too. The source of protein in the powder is important. Soy and whey are common proteins and both can create dampness. A better source is pea protein. Peas are legumes, but in powder form they are stripped of their gift of fiber that aids digestion. Protein powder smoothies can create problems for the stomach. When we drink a cold smoothie, there is a gush of cold fluid that is hard to digest, especially if there is any sweetener in the powder. Over time, this habit creates internal dampness for the digestive system. The stomach does best with warm cooked foods that we chew and drinks that are body temperature.

### What about carbonation?

Carbonated drinks are dehydrating! The more carbonated beverages you consume, the more thirsty you will become. Please avoid carbonated beverages, they are very big problems for the stomach and digestive tract, even seltzer water!

### How about drinking coffee?

Coffee is considered bitter and energetically very warming, even iced coffee is energetically warming to the body, although the ice makes it very cold to the stomach. The caffeine in coffee revs up the kidney energy (think: adrenal glands), and it also stimulates the heart. When we drink too much coffee, we may actually experience the heart beat racing. A little coffee, like one occasional cup in the morning, may nourish the heart because the heart needs the bitter flavor.  The heart and kidneys have a relationship, they try to balance each other. When we drink too  much coffee, and we experience a rush of energy,  the rush does not nourish the heart's or the kidneys' energy. It is like revving up the car engine, but going nowhere while consuming energy. Our poor heart qi and kidney qi! It is exhausting for the heart and kidneys to go through the ups and downs of too much caffeine every day, over time. If the coffee has sweetener and dairy products in it (cream or milk), it is very sticky for the stomach to handle. Sugar, dairy, and gluten are the stickiest foods we can eat. This means they are particularly difficult to digest — they create a sluggishness in the digestive tract, leading to internal dampness or other problems.

### OK, tea must be better, right?

Tea is a little different from coffee. Although there is some caffeine in tea, there is much less compared to coffee. There are many varieties of tea (green, oolong, black, and white), but in general, tea is cooling to the body, especially green tea. Tea lifts the energy (qi) in the body to brighten the mind. It also lightens the qi for the stomach, it is a digestive helper. Of course, too much of anything is not helpful. How much is too much? That depends on what is needed at that time in order to create balance in your own stomach and body.

Herbal "teas" are actually infusions. They are not made from tea leaves, but from other herbs such as chamomile or peppermint. We will explore some herbs used for cooking in the recipe section, and many of the same herbs make very nice infusions. Remember every plant has an energetic property that we take in when we drink (or eat) that herb. For example, peppermint is very cooling, so drinking peppermint tea will cool your stomach. Ginger is very warming, so generally drinking ginger tea will warm your stomach. Drinking warm beverages, even hot water, has a warming effect in the body.

### What does Chinese Medicine say about alcohol?

Alcohol is worth mentioning. It has been researched that a small amount (1-2 oz) of plum wine or sherry before dinner may be an appetizer, meaning may stimulate the appetite. A glass of red wine helps the blood move (circulation), and is also heating the stomach. Another way of saying this is that the pH of alcohol is acidic (hot) and the accumulation of heat in the stomach over time destroys digestive health, and the health of the blood vessels. The stomach functions optimally at body temperature. Too much heat or too little heat from what we ingest can hinder our stomach's ability to digest. For example, if you tend to eat red meat and very few vegetables and drink alcohol, this is a very "hot" diet. If you eat only vegetables and no dairy (a vegan diet), this a "cool" diet, and you may need to warm up the stomach a bit for good health.

Alcohol can contribute to our happy experiences in life; and alcohol can powerfully destroy happiness in life. This is not an easy drink to balance for much of humanity. As always, the advice of TCM is to go the middle way, no extremes; and always consider what is needed in order to create balance within.

### Drink water!

In short, the best thing to drink is water— hot, warm or cool, not iced. Second best may be green tea. Juices and alcohol are to be imbibed in small amounts, occasionally, or never.

NOTE: In the Appendix section of this book, there is a detailed discussion of the TCM understanding of the digestive process called The Energetics of Digestion (pg.112).

"Sugar, dairy, and gluten are the stickiest foods we can eat. This means they are particularly difficult to digest."

# Food Is Energy: Another Dimension of Eating

Satisfaction from eating is derived from being fully present while eating your food. It may sound simple, but this is easier said than done.

The way to establish a healthy relationship with food is to connect with your body. Connecting with the body is the first practice of Zhineng Qigong (pronounced chee-gong) — and it is a practice not just for eating, but for living life! When we are connected with our body, our mind is focused inside the body. Usually, we are focused on the external world via our five senses — how we look, what car we drive, money — in short, our appearance in the world. This orientation can feel competitive and make us lose ourselves and what we think matters to advertising, our culture, the virtual world, or the people we associate with. When our mind is focused externally it leads to many problems. When we bring our attention inside our body, our busy mind comes home, home to ourselves in our body. It is necessary for our mind to come home to our body in order for healing to happen, and nourishing ourselves is a form of healing. Through practice, coming home to our body and connecting deep inside becomes so comfortable and pleasant that we don't want to ever lose our connection to ourselves, even in daily life.

How do you do it? Close your eyes, relax by taking deep, slow breaths, and notice all sensations and feelings inside your body. Take some time practicing this. Then softly open your eyes, staying connected to your experience of yourself inside. Do this while choosing your food at the grocery store, in the garden, or from your pantry. Connect with your body while you're preparing and cooking your food — and, especially, as you eat your food. (NOTE: See "Cooking and Eating as Meditation," pg. 26 for detailed guidance).

Note that this practice is very different from using your analytical mind to select food and to know about nutrition, and to know about the digestion process. Embodied eating means that we perceive everything as energy! That's right: Food is energy. Your body is energy. Your digestive system integrating the food with the body is an energetic integration. Astrophysics has proven that formless energy makes up 96% of the Universe; and we know that 99.9% of our human body is energy (called electron clouds) yet, this knowledge is still unincorporated into daily life. Coming home to our body is the beginning practice for **experiencing** our own energy and from there going on to experience the energy in the Universe!

Connect with your body and connect with nature. Nature supplies the variety of flavors and colors and seasons which produce the variety of tastes and qualities in your food. By strengthening our digestive system energy, we are better able to digest the food we eat. Eating a variety of foods is best for the body. This includes a variety of tastes: sweet, salty, sour, bitter, spicy, and pungent. And a variety of colors of food: green, red, yellow, orange, blue, purple, white, brown, and black. Nothing we eat or need comes from outside of our planet earth. We are intimately, energetically connected to each other and to life on planet earth. This realization brings us to a place of gratitude — we are grateful for nature and for our physical existence. Deeply, we are grateful that there is energy and we can experience it!

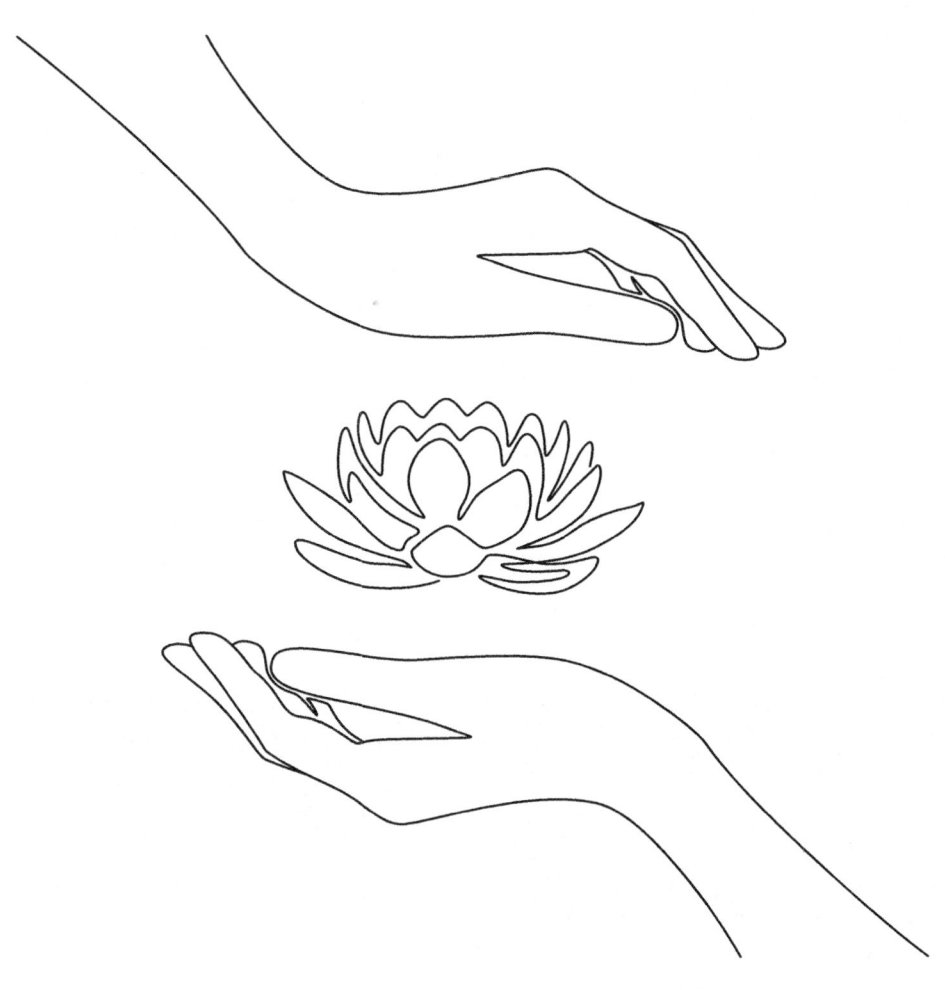

Embodied eating means that we perceive
everything as energy!

# Cooking & Eating as Meditation

There are many ways to meditate. Meditation is such an ancient practice, found in some form in every major world religion. Why is it so prevalent for all people all over the world? Maybe meditation is a time-honored way to assist us in our search for answers to our questions in life. Meditation is a means for tuning into ourselves and to the living Universe. A paradox, perhaps, but both the mystery of ourselves (Who am I?) and the mystery of The Universe (What is life all about?) are part of the human experience. Recognition of the health benefits of meditation are well researched and growing. Meditation may also be an approach to spiritual cultivation.

I practice and am offering a meditation form where we deeply connect inside our own body, especially to our heart. We value our body as the means by which we experience our precious human life, and develop our qi and consciousness. All aspects of being human are respected, no single part of us needs to be avoided or "walled off." It is good to be fully human, that is what we are here to be. Therefore, learning how to meditate inside of our body is valued. We recognize the heart as the home of our human spirit. Heart-to-heart communication and heart-to-heart connections are the most satisfying and nourishing level of human relationships. Connecting with our own heart is a skillful means to cultivating a joyful, healthy relationship with ourselves — and then with others and life! We cannot separate our body, our energy, and our consciousness. However, whichever of these we focus on is how we will cultivate ourselves. When we feel stuck, repeating thoughts or stories of our life, or feelings, our energy gets stuck. Over time, stuck energy creates blocked energy, and  blocked energy creates health problems.

This is a gradual process. First we learn how to relax and come in to our body. Then we learn how to experience our qi. Then we practice opening to and cultivating our deep pure consciousness, our True Self. Thank goodness that there are stable, ancient practices and teachers to guide us if we choose to develop ourselves along this path.

The purpose of meditating and cooking — and meditating and eating — is to deeply relax our body and mind for the benefit of our health. We cannot experience our energy when we are stressed out and going very fast internally. Learning how to relax and tune into ourselves is the first step in increasing our awareness. From a relaxed state, we may experience our qi and gain more awareness. The more awareness we have, the more in touch we feel with ourselves and with the living Universe, the more emotional stability and physical health we cultivate. This is important on the path of spiritual development (also called increasing consciousness).

**Making Your Own Guided Meditation for Cooking & Eating**

I suggest reading the following script out loud and making a recording for yourself to practice with. Read slowly, pausing between sentences, so you find your own pace when you use your recording for guided meditation. Don't be surprised if you need to revise your recordings as time goes by, growing slower and slower. Maybe this is a measure of your nervous system calming down, getting more relaxed, so that it becomes a welcome pleasure to slow down for a few minutes each day! You may listen to the recording as a guide for meditation both before you prepare to cook and during cooking!

Allow the recorded words to assist you in relaxing. This way you don't need to use focused thinking to remember what to do! When we meditate this way, we use a different part of the brain from the part we use when reading and concentrating. We want to be free to focus internally, and not have our attention move back and forth from meditating to reading instructions. As you practice, this will become more fluid and comfortable. Playfully enjoy this as a process of discovery and adventure.

You may experience yourself in deeper connection with who you are and with your heart. Then, you can bring this wisdom to your food. You may be tuning into your ingredients in a new way, and appreciating the life that is nourishing your life in a new way. You may experience something different each time you cook this way. When we connect with ourselves, we may find how dynamic we truly are, developing an active awareness with our loving, kind heart, the residence of our human spirit, deep inside. This is a path of deep transformation into a happy, beautiful life!

"Smile into your day."

# Cooking & Eating Meditation Script

"Before cooking or eating, either standing or sitting or lying down, close your eyes and feel your heart inside your chest. Slowing down your busy mind by focusing inside your body. Coming "home" inside your body. Nowhere else to be right now, nothing else to do right now; allowing a few precious minutes for relaxing, regrouping, and slowing down. Merging your attention into your heart and relaxing. Taking some slow, deep breaths and relaxing into your heart even more. Feeling connected to your heart, allowing it to gently open inside, open to yourself. Breathing. Smiling. Smiling on your lips and smiling inside your heart. Noticing all sensations and emotions inside of your body. Simply noticing — no need to do anything, no need to analyze, evaluate, nor change anything — just allowing whatever you are noticing.

Now begin relaxing and smiling into your entire body. Relaxing and softening the muscles in your face, especially around your eyes and nose and mouth. Breathing and letting go of any tension in your shoulders and neck. Relaxing your upper arms and elbows, relaxing your lower arms and wrists. Feeling relaxation spreading in your hands, your palms, and your fingers. Now, moving your attention to your back; slowly, gently breathing relaxation into your entire back, letting go of any tension. Now breathing relaxation into your chest and abdomen, taking as much time as you need, relaxing more and more. Now releasing tension in your hips, and down your legs. Softly breathing and relaxing your upper legs, knees, lower legs, and ankles. Relaxing your feet, the soles of your feet and toes releasing any tension. Feeling your feet relaxing. Gently, softly breathing into your entire body, feeling comfortable in your own skin, continuously releasing any tension.

If you are noticing any areas of discomfort, gently breathing and smiling into those areas, without resisting or struggling against sensations in your body. Deeply allowing what you are noticing, including areas of comfort and areas of discomfort. Deeply accepting whatever you may be noticing inside. Continuously relaxing. Recognizing any areas of discomfort as energy that is not flowing, energy that is stuck. And recognizing any areas of comfort as energy that is freely flowing. Qi is neither "good" nor "bad" — qi is either stuck or flowing. Relaxing and noticing "what is" inside, more and more. As you are breathing into areas of discomfort, noticing and allowing any sensation you find there; and noticing that the sensations may be softening, may be easing, may be disappearing as you are gently accepting whatever you are experiencing. Being very patient with yourself. Do not force anything, never forcing your qi; just relaxing and allowing yourself to experience your qi. Allowing yourself to learn from your energy, as you experience yourself inwardly, in this moment.

Now gently, slowly breathe from the center of your body, from inside your lower abdomen, between your navel and low back. Inhaling upward. Visualizing and feeling each breath moving from the center of your lower abdomen upward, inside of you, toward your heart, so easy, so relaxing. Exhaling gently, letting go of any effort, noticing and allowing qi floating downward again to the center of your body. Relaxing with each cycle of breath. Inhaling *from the lower abdomen center upward, and exhaling, letting go and relaxing back downward. So easy, so comfortable, so relaxing. Enjoying the sensation of this simple breathing. Meditate this way for as long as you like. Feeling your breath lifting toward your heart.*

—PAUSE—

*Now feeling inside your heart. Relaxing and breathing gently, connecting and smiling into your heart. It's as if you are sitting inside your heart, experiencing your big heart, and with every breath, your heart's energy is opening and expanding. Very simply breathing and relaxing and merging into your heart. Allowing all sensations, continuously relaxing and noticing deep inside. You may experience your heart's energy opening up, maybe bigger than your physical heart. Gently noticing this, and allowing all sensations; nothing to aim for, nothing to achieve, nothing to miss out on, simply connecting with and experiencing your own heart and its energy. Who is connecting and experiencing your heart? Your internal observer is merging with your heart's energy. When this happens, your pure consciousness recognizes itself and awakens! There is no separation between your inner observer and heart, you are completely merged, as one. The heart's consciousness wakes up and this state is your True Self. You are not observing yourself as if you are outside of yourself. You are completely immersed in the present moment in pure consciousness, your consciousness aware of itself, connected with your True Self, your heart.*

*If thoughts, emotions, or other distracting sensations arise, notice them and go deeper than the sensations or feelings or thoughts, deeper into your heart. Staying connected to your heart and not to the thoughts, emotions, or sensations. Emotions are like ocean waves, they come and go, often with a story and a lot of movement on the surface. Dive under the waves of emotion, connect with your pure consciousness underneath the feelings and allow the loving wisdom of the heart to transform your experience. Your heart's consciousness knows how to do this without any instructions. Go beyond thinking, relax into your True Self, into your pure consciousness.*

*Your mind cannot approach or heal emotions in the same, effective way as your heart. Allowing yourself the possibility of experiencing the capacity of your heart. Continuously breathing and resting inside of your heart for as long as you like."*

—PAUSE—

When you are ready to end meditation time, slowly and gently focus on your physical body, again noticing all sensations and emotions, and begin moving your body, stretching as needed, returning to normal consciousness, and slowly opening your eyes. Now take a moment to stay connected to yourself, your heart, with your eyes open before getting up.

## Meditating While Cooking/Cooking Embodied

If you are cooking, practice whatever your next task is with a connection to your heart. Can you relax and feel your heart's energy? Can you chop and stir, feeling your energy moving through your arms and hands from your heart? You may experience some tingling, or a sensation like your hands are enlarged, or warm. Again, nothing that you "should" feel, just allowing for the development of awareness of your qi. Can you feel a lightness, a joyousness from your heart? Regardless of external circumstances, can you allow the joy that is the nature of the heart to prevail? Enjoy yourself and the pleasure of cooking and creating. Stay relaxed, focused, and joyful during cooking. You will taste the energy from this practice in your food!

Every time you practice meditating, meeting yourself this way, it will be a different experience. This method of connecting inside helps us to relax our body and emotions. We practice experiencing our own energy and accepting our own energy as we find it, in the present moment. We practice connecting with our heart, the home of our human spirit. Our pure consciousness grows. Through regular practice, you may develop your capacity to not only connect with your heart but to live your life guided by the wisdom and joy residing inside your heart. If this is of interest to you, I suggest finding a Heart-Centered Meditation teacher or Zhineng Qigong pure consciousness teacher to help guide you. It is the most spiritually rewarding path, and also the most challenging one, when we truly encounter ourselves and our limitations, and learn to go beyond the "thinking mind" to meet your True Self.

## Meditating While Eating/Eating Embodied

When you are eating, here is an experiment you may like to try, I call it "embodied eating." First, sitting at the dinner table with your plate of delicious food, bring your attention home to your body by practicing the meditation introduced above. Now from very deeply connecting with yourself, take a bite of food and chew with your eyes closed. Chew until there is nothing left in your mouth, really sensing the food. What do you notice about your food? What do you notice about the flavors and textures of the food? How does the food make you feel, both physically and emotionally? Reflect on the life history of the food — did it grow wild? Did it roam or swim free? Was it showered with clean water or chemical herbicides? Think about what it is bringing to your body. Ask yourself: How was the food cooked? Was it steamed? If so, it will bring moisture. Was it grilled? If so, it will bring fiery heat. Was the food carefully, lovingly prepared? Remember, you are taking in, eating, all of these qualities of these energies. Stay very connected to your own experience, this is how we sense a connection with our food.

This practice provides an opportunity to appreciate your food and your body in a profound way! After continuous practice, your nervous system will begin to respond, too. You are training yourself to relax, slow down, connect with yourself and enjoy the present moment, and enjoy life in a simple and yet very satisfying way. The result can be improved digestive health, better mental and emotional health, a calmed nervous system, even improved sleep — and more healing. You may begin to become more simple in food choices and in everyday living. If you allow yourself to open up to the wisdom inside your body, inside every organ and cell, you will experience life in a truly embodied way!

# How to Live a Happy Life - From the Heart

The heart is multi-dimensional. Physically, it circulates blood. Emotionally, it is where happiness and joy come from. Mentally, it influences how we perceive and think. And it is also the residence of our human spirit which circulates throughout our body. When we cultivate a lifestyle connected with our heart's energy, we are better able to live a happy life. We may see the quality of the heart/spirit reflected in a person's eyes.

Integrating our human spirit into our daily living creates happiness and health. In fact, scientific research has proven that laughter facilitates healing. That means there is a direct correlation between a joyful heart and healing. But how do we develop a joyful heart and live a happy life?

This is a general guide for people of any faith or wisdom tradition. Feel free to insert your own spiritual vocabulary wherever it applies. The purpose of this guide is to help cultivate our human spirit, via the heart, as a vital component of our health and happiness.

According to Traditional Chinese Medicine, there are three resources available to us during this human existence. We call them the Three Treasures:

- **The physical (Jing) resource:** Jing is the energy that funds an individual's physical life — the body, its growth and development, DNA and hormones, vitality and longevity.
- **The energy (Qi) resource:** Qi is the energy that funds the creation and operation of all life. It condenses into form and creates the body and all matter. And it disperses into a formless, ever-present state in the Universe. In the body, Qi is produced by the stomach and pancreas/spleen and has different qualities depending on its location and function.
- **The consciousness (Shen) resource:** Shen is the energy of consciousness. It is the awareness of the emotional, mental, and spiritual dimensions of being human. The heart is the residence of Shen. Consciousness can be cultivated, and the Shen reflects our spiritual cultivation.

"Your heart is lovingly waiting for you to connect with it."

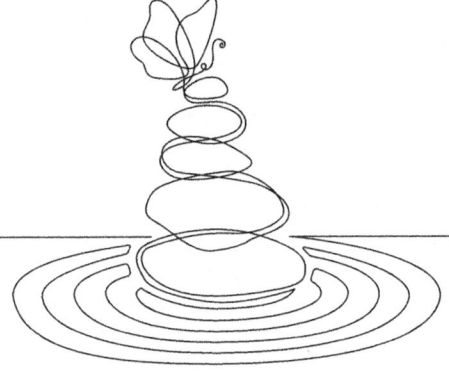

Jing, Qi, and Shen are interconnected with each other, they influence one another. If your Jing is healthy and your Qi is flowing, then your Shen will be healthy and happy. If your Shen is strong and clear, then your Qi and Jing will improve. Hopefully in this lifetime, we work to attune and increase our awareness of, and experience with, all Three Treasures. Access to the Three Treasures is located inside of our human body. Perhaps one purpose of life is to become fully human, to experience living embodied and fully connected to our heart.

Living embodied and connected to our heart is a pathway to personal development, stronger relationships, better health, and more joy. On the flip side, living disconnected from our body and our heart leads to many difficulties physically, socially, psychologically, and spiritually.

To give order to our day is to give order to our thoughts. Here are some basic suggestions to help you plan your day in order to develop your heart, which in turn, cultivates both happiness — and good health.

## Morning: Awakening the Heart

In the morning, energy is open for a new day. It's our opportunity to open ourselves to our energy. Upon awakening and before getting out of bed, be grateful for another day of life! Smile into your day. Then, get out of bed, breathe deeply and begin moving your body. Keep your conscious attention on your movement **inside** your body, allowing your qi to flow. (Mimic stretching like your pet does each time they wake up!) Dedicate your day to the highest benefit for all life.

Next, so you can allow life's energy to freely flow, focus on the entry into your home (feng shui). Clear any obstacles from the front or main door and clean the entry area, so qi is free to circulate into your home, nourishing all who live there.

Then, move on to cleaning yourself — internally and externally. When we have a practice that focuses us internally — via qigong or yoga or breath work or martial arts or meditation or prayer — we are moving our energy and being truly embodied. This is an internal cleanse activating jing and qi. These methods boost and encourage more qi to flow within you, which can increase your capacity to enjoy life, cultivating shen. Then shower or bathe, cleaning the outside of your body.

Next, eat some breakfast (grain and protein) and drink some warm tea, perhaps practicing "embodied eating."

We choose what food we eat in order to create health. Likewise, we may carefully choose what information we take in to create happiness and health.

What if you were to look at your phone at this point in the morning, instead of first thing? How will you respond to what you read on your phone? This is the "real-life" application of your daily practice. Once again, smile into your heart and breathe. Remember that you are perfectly designed for your life. You can handle what comes your way — and energy is moving and transforming continuously in life as well as within you. Try it, see how you feel for the entire day! Now you are ready to go out into the world with a more peaceful, happy heart.

## Through the Day: Living Through the Heart

As you move through your day, what if you inwardly wish for the highest benefit for yourself and for anyone you encounter? Make this intention gently, happily, breathing with it. Wherever you are going — whether driving, riding a subway, bus, bicycle, or walking — return your mind to your heart and wish the highest good for anyone you pass. How does this influence your attitude? Does it stir any part of you? Just notice inside. Smile externally and/or internally toward yourself and your fellow human beings.

What if you extend your thoughts into actions — look for ways to be kind? It may be as simple as opening a door for someone or sincerely thanking a person for their assistance. Notice how good it feels to offer kindness and assistance to someone else.

Everyone is struggling somehow in life, this is the nature of life. When we encounter our limitations, we feel uncomfortable, unsure of ourselves or how to proceed. This is by design so that we recognize our need to learn - to outgrow our current ways! So acknowledge others' humanity as you acknowledge your own humanity. We are all people with feelings, concerns, and personal issues, all wanting happiness — in this regard we are all the same. Keeping this in mind keeps your heart's wisdom at the forefront, not needing to justify your thoughts and actions. You can stay connected to your inner wisdom and loving-kindness this way. When you notice getting distracted from this intention, simply and gently return to it by smiling inside your heart.

How much do you laugh during your day? Laughing is so good for health and wellbeing! Even if you cannot find anything to laugh about, practice laughing just for yourself. You may pretend to laugh until you find yourself enjoying the silliness of it all — and eventually you will laugh genuinely. Laughing relaxes the heart, and when the heart relaxes, we laugh more easily. Practice laughing for a few minutes each day, as your own meditation practice!

My mother's advice for everyone was to have at least one big belly laugh each day. She created her own sunshine by doing this, even when life got very challenging!

## Evening: Resting the Heart

When you return home, there are practices to help close the day. You might begin by cooking and eating with embodied energy. This helps to bring about a more peaceful, happy heart and you simply feel better. (NOTE: Use the suggested meditation script and guidelines on pg. 26). As a result, our relationships improve. This is a powerful practice!

When the chores of the day are finished, spend a few minutes gently reflecting — noticing your interactions with others, forgiving others and yourself, and having "the attitude of infinite gratitude" for your precious life. Maybe practice meditation, or pray, or read inspiring wisdom books, or listen to teachings by loving, wisdom teachers. I had a friend in Japan whose father would often invite a local poet or philosopher to his home in the evening for tea, quiet discussion, and sharing. It was a way for him to cultivate his human spirit.

Whatever your practice may be, always rest your mind and heart on good, beautiful, positive information. Before sleeping, clean yourself (brush your teeth, wash your face or whole body), and then go to bed.

In preparation for sleep, practice relaxing your entire body deeply so the body gets trained to let go of any tension. In this way, your mind and heart also let go of any tension and your quality of sleep improves. All this, again, leads to improving your quality of life.

**Heart-Conscious, Happy Living Takes Practice**

It's pretty easy to intellectually understand these suggestions for daily life. And yet, it may be very challenging to actually put into practice! Emotional and physical obstacles can arise that might be surprising and difficult. Take heart, and continue practicing!

It can be helpful to find a well-qualified, experienced guide for your heart and happiness journey — as well as spiritual friends. Be cautious to protect your tender heart as it becomes stronger and stronger.

Naturally, you may have times when you are disciplined and dedicated to your practice, and other times when you get distracted from it. When you recognize you've fallen away from your consciousness cultivation practice, simply and gently return to it! That is all you can do, and it is a lot!

Your heart is so benevolent. It is patiently, lovingly waiting for you to connect with it — and it will be there for you, your entire life.

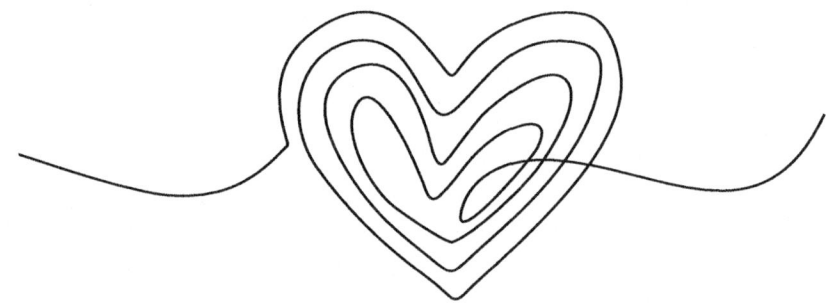

"Now you are ready to go out into the world with a more peaceful, happy heart."

# recipes

The recipes in this book are not divided by breakfast, lunch, and dinner — or by main dishes, side dishes, and desserts. Instead, they are organized into three sections:

## Yuan, Ying, and Wei

These are levels that Traditional Chinese Medicine uses to describe where our food comes from and how it influences the body. As you learn which foods belong in each level, you will better understand the energetic healing qualities of food.

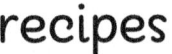

# yuan recipes

Recipes in the Yuan section focus on ingredients
that mostly come from the waters.

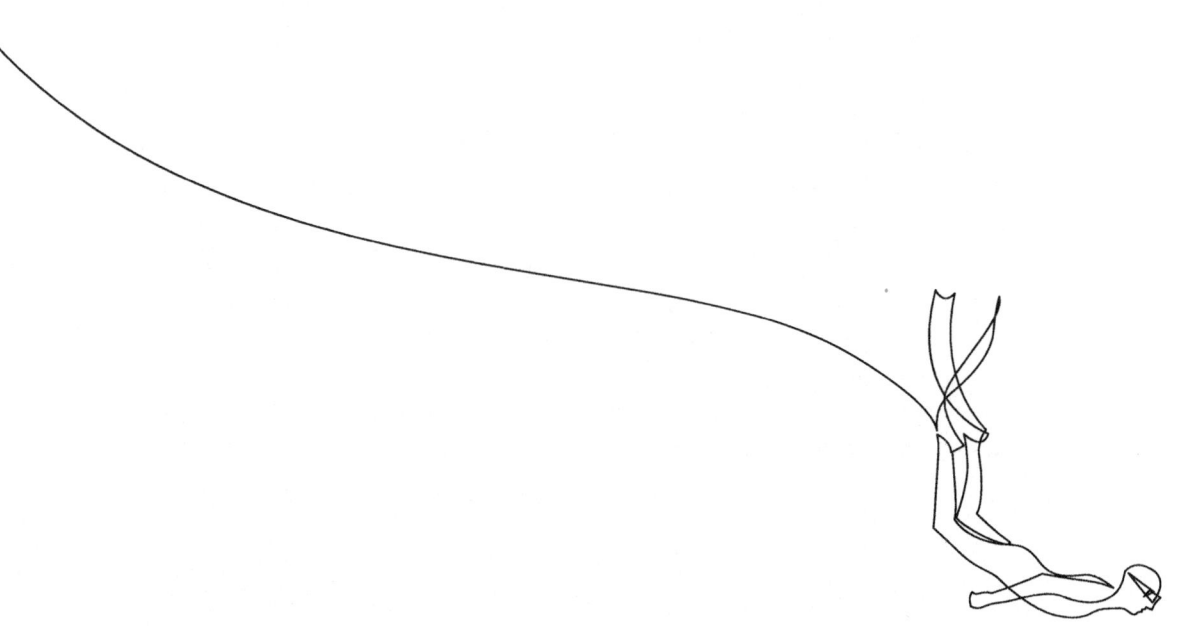

# Broiled Salmon

**Serves 3-6** | **Cook time: 10-15 minutes**

*This is a simple dish and an example of the food and the cooking method balancing each other. And a quick tip on cooking fish: Overcooking fish ruins its amazing flavor. This is often the reason a lot of folks think they don't care for fish!*

## INGREDIENTS

1-2 lbs. fresh Salmon, with skin on
olive oil
salt
lemon (optional)

## DIRECTIONS

NOTE: It's best to use a cast iron griddle or skillet, the iron subtly infuses whatever you cook on it, nourishing blood.

Wash the fish.

Pour a little olive oil on the skillet and gently rub a little olive oil on the skin of the salmon.

Place the salmon flesh side down, skin side up, on the skillet.

Turn the oven on broil, and place the skillet on the highest oven shelf setting, directly under the broiling elements.

Cook until the skin gets brown/black and shrinks and curls around the edges, about 5 minutes or less.

Remove the skillet from the oven and scrape off the darkened skin.

Salt the fish and gently flip it over.

Put it back in the oven to broil for another minute or two, until the flesh is warmed through, but not dry and flaky.

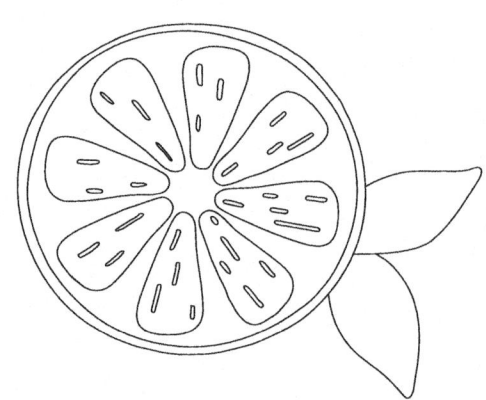

**Salmon** — This fish swims in both fresh water and ocean water, which is quite remarkable! Because it lives in the water, it brings us the water element in its nourishment. It supports kidney energy. Kidney energy nourishes the bones, hormone system, especially the reproductive system, and of course, water in the body (urination system).

**Broiling** — This process can be considered a fire element method of cooking, bringing heat quickly into the food.

**Balance** — Because this recipe combines both fire and water elements, they balance each other.

Too much fire, and the water element dries up; too much water puts out the fire element. A perfect balance of these elements means that a tempered fire and warmed water mutually support each other, and therefore nourish and balance our body the same way.

To make this recipe into a complete meal, remember the formula is grain, green, and protein! Cook some rice, saute some chard or kale or another green vegetable, and you have a basic meal. Add more vegetables, such as yellow vegetables (butternut squash, yellow squash, etc.) and you've increased the nutrients to your meal. So quick and easy and good!

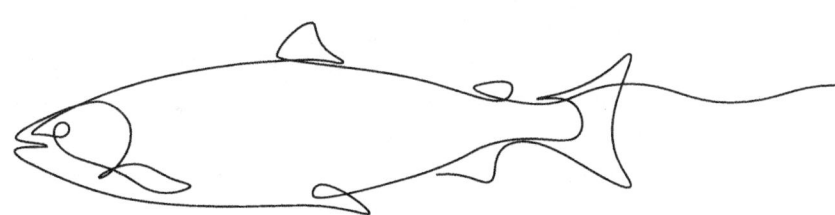

# Smoked Trout (or Salmon) w/Warm Potato Salad

**Serves 4-6  |  Cook time: 45 minutes**

*This is a good recipe for a fall day when the apples are freshly picked and in the market. The trout is a little harder to find in the store, so you may also substitute with smoked salmon. I often serve it with some fresh green beans to complete this meal.*

## INGREDIENTS

2 tbsp. salt-cured capers
2 lbs. baby red or gold potatoes
8 ounces smoked trout (or salmon)
olive oil
lemon juice
pepper
1 tart Granny Smith apple
1 tbsp. fresh dill

## DIRECTIONS

Soak the capers in water and rinse them after 10 minutes of soaking.
Boil the potatoes, uncovered, until tender (about 20 minutes), then drain.
Break trout (or salmon) into bite-sized pieces.
Wash, core, and slice the apple into very thin slices.
Set a 1-quart pan over medium-high heat, and add ⅓ c. olive oil.
When the oil ripples, add the capers (it will splatter, stand back!).
Stir capers until the berries have opened, about 1 minute.
Pour capers into a fine wire strainer over a glass measuring cup and reserve the oil.
Drain the capers on a paper towel.
In a large serving bowl, whisk the oil from the capers with ¼ c. lemon juice and pepper.
Stir in the potatoes.
Add the smoked trout (or salmon), apple and dill.
Sprinkle the capers over the top and serve.

This recipe has a little bit of everything! My teacher in Japan said that every dinner should have the 4 main food groups:

**Air** — tree nuts, fruits, or birds

**Ground** — plants or animals

**Below the ground** — root vegetables

**Sea** — fish, seaweeds, or sea vegetables

(This Japanese system is slightly different from the Chinese system of 3 levels — Yuan, Ying, and Wei).

**Potatoes** — White potatoes nourish the stomach, pancreas/spleen. They are cooling for heat in the blood (high blood pressure, high cholesterol). Because they are cooling, you may slice raw potato and put it on burns on the skin to help heal and soothe the burns. The green leaves, skin, and roots of potatoes are toxic.

*Note: Normally, I don't combine fruit with other foods, as it does not digest well. However, when it is used to tenderize meats, it is a good thing. The combination of the tart apple and the oil and trout (or salmon), with the acidic lemon balances well and is easy to digest. This is another dish kids and adults both enjoy.*

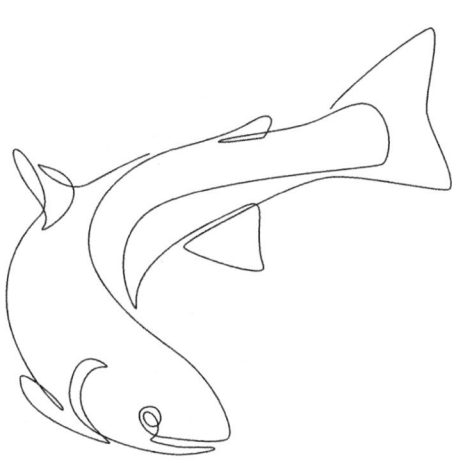

# Spinach Rice with Shrimp

**Serves 4-6  |  Cook time: 30-40 minutes**

*The ideal meal includes a whole grain, vegetables, and protein. This is a Mediterranean dish that is a complete and ideal meal by itself. This dish combines rice, spinach, onion, tomato sauce, and some herbs, with shrimp. When my children were in their growth-spurt years, I cooked this using chicken broth instead of water, just for added protein. Usually, water is all that is needed to cook the rice and vegetables. It is delicious!*

## INGREDIENTS

2 bunches of fresh spinach — washed, dried, chopped
2-4 tbsp. olive oil
1 small onion, minced
1 garlic clove, minced
2 tsp. fresh parsley, chopped
2 tsp. dried oregano
1 c. uncooked rice
1 (8-ounce) can tomato sauce
2 c. water
salt and pepper to taste
1 lb. large shrimp, cleaned

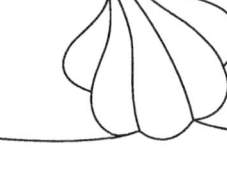

Optional:
¼ c. butter, ½ a stick)
feta cheese, crumbled
2 c. chicken broth, instead of 2 c. water

## DIRECTIONS

Wash and dry the spinach, and cut into small pieces and set aside.
Sauté, in olive oil, the onion, garlic, and oregano in a sauté pan over medium heat.
Add the rice and slightly brown all the ingredients together.
Add the tomato sauce and water and bring to a boil, adding salt and pepper to taste.
Once the rice is cooking, add the spinach and parsley and cook for 15 minutes.
Lastly, add the shrimp and cook for 5 minutes.
Gently place the meal in a serving dish and enjoy!

If you are including dairy products in this dish you may brown the butter and pour it over the shrimp. After the food is in a serving dish, you may sprinkle some feta cheese on top.

**Shrimp** — Shrimp brings the Yuan level of food to this meal. Shrimp, a crustacean, is considered more Yang energy, moving around the ocean with legs. Fish do not have legs, they swim, so they are considered less Yang than crustaceans. Sea creatures that do not move around on their own, like clams (shell dwellers), are the most Yin of the relatively Yin seafood category. The stillness of clams and the water environment are more Yin qualities.

**Spinach** — the leaves spread out and up, corresponding to liver/gallbladder. spinach is cooling and moves qi downward.

**Onion/Garlic** — these are very hot, stimulating foods. Use them carefully and infrequently in cooking. They are also dehydrating.

**Rice** — is a grain that strongly supports Stomach, Pancreas, Spleen. White rice is hydrating, protecting Stomach yin (the lining of the Stomach organ).

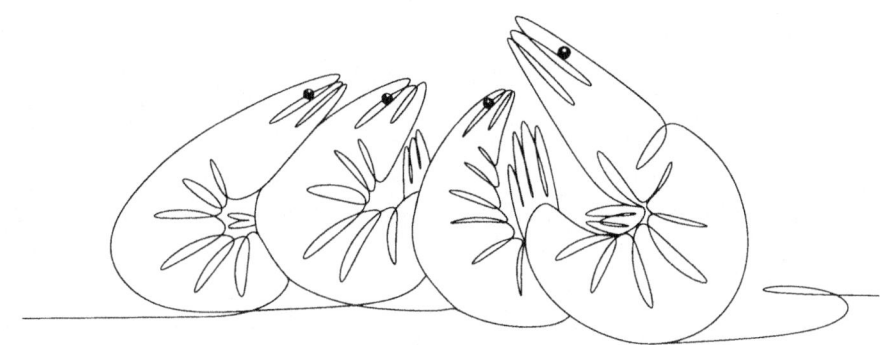

# Sauteed Mushrooms

**Serves 4-6  |  Cook time: 15-30 minutes**

*The only difficulty with mushrooms is cleaning them. Soaking mushrooms also helps them to loosen the dirt, and to rehydrate them if they look tired. You may buy dehydrated mushrooms and soak them back to their elegant form. Different species of mushrooms have very different flavors and textures and shapes. Be adventurous and try as many varieties as you can! It is so easy to cook mushrooms once you have cleaned them and cut off the ragged bottom of their stems. Do include the stem and enjoy them along with the "top cap" of the mushroom. Eat them on their own or add them to almost any vegetable for an earthy flavor and damp absorbing function.*

## INGREDIENTS

1 lb. of mushrooms, sliced
1 tbsp. olive oil
1 tbsp. butter
1 pinch of sea salt

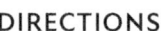

## DIRECTIONS

Warm the oils in a sauté pan.
Add the mushrooms with a pinch of salt.
Turn the mushrooms while they shrink and cook in the pan.

Some people prefer their mushrooms barely cooked, still absorbent. Others prefer them more well-cooked, harder to bite. Experiment to find your own taste. You may also combine various species of mushrooms together. Personally, I love sautéed mushrooms and chard, and a bowl of rice, for lunch!

---

CHINESE MEDICINE REFERENCES

**Mushrooms** — They grow in dark, moist places. They consume the dampness of their environment and transform it into their being. Therefore, mushrooms are considered helpful to dry dampness in the digestive system. They are a fungus, and absorb fungal growths in the body.

**Sea salt** — Has an affinity to the kidneys, and tastes different depending on where it's from. Grey sea salt comes from the Celtic Sea or France, and tastes wonderful! Land salt is pink from the Himalayas. Kosher salt has large crystals. Use iodized salt only if you do not eat seaweed or fish.

# ying recipes

Recipes in the Ying section focus on ingredients that come from the land.
This is where most of our food comes from.

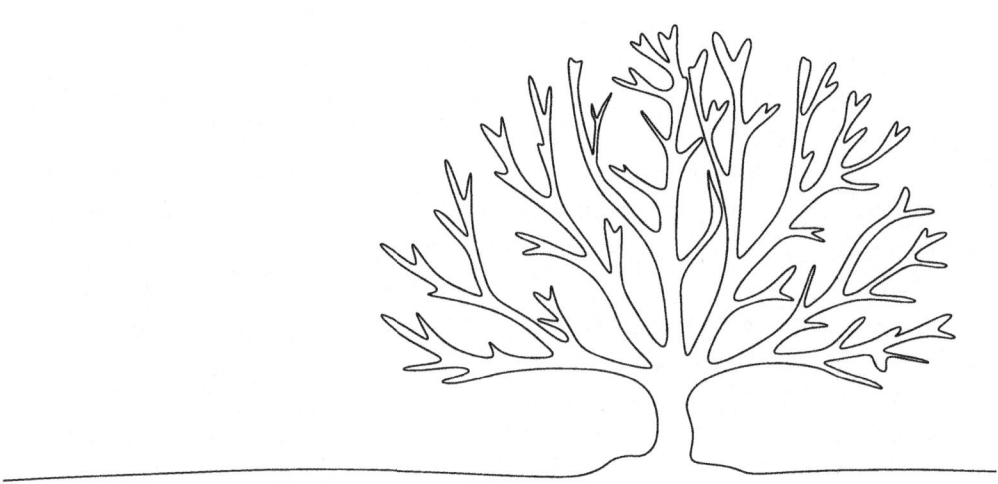

**Thinking about the energetics of food**

*This recipe was the first one I wrote for this book. Its story was the inspiration for communicating the feeling of using food for healing in the energetic sense. Can you read the story and sense the energy of the environment, the intention, the food selection — all consciously chosen to achieve the healing capacity of the ingredients? Somehow, I couldn't shorten the way this original story came together with the recipe. It captures the essence of this book, of the entirety — the physical, emotional, energetic, and consciousness embodied in food!*

# Chicken Soup

Serves 4-6  |  Cook time: 1 hour

*It's late afternoon and snowing. Yesterday my neighbor died at home, his wife told me in a state of shock. So, the most healing, soothing thing I can think of is to bring her a pot of chicken soup. It really is healing food.*

*Chicken is considered the earth bird, as it supports the earth energy inside us. That's short-hand for creating harmony, stability, and strength in our stomach and digestive tract. It also nourishes our immune system, just what we need when we are facing challenging times.*

*Today I'm taking a shortcut and using a baked chicken from the grocery store deli. My time is limited, so I'm happy for the convenience of the roasted chicken.*

*First, remove the skin and separate the bones from the flesh. I put the skin and bones in a pot of water, water just covering the chicken remains. Then allow the heat from the water to soak up the goodness from the chicken.*

*Bones store our Jing energy. This is the essence energy of the body, where our marrow, blood, and thus, DNA is stored. Jing has to do with the vital energy of our life force. When we replenish this Jing through eating bones (and making soup from bones is an easy way to accomplish this), we are creating and fostering support for our kidneys' energy system, which supports our immune system.*

*Chicken is also a warming meat, and just right to eat on a cold day. The warmth within the meat balances the cold temperature outside, which supports our immune system, too. Balance is a healthy state in Chinese Medicine. "Balance" means the food brings a state of harmony to the body, for that person at that particular time. There is no "balanced" diet for all people, rather there is creating balance within each person. And what is "balancing" to eat at one time, may not achieve balance at another time, depending on our age, environment, state of health — physically, emotionally, mentally, and spiritually.*

*Back to my soup. While the bones and skin are boiling, I sauté carrots, onions, and celery in olive oil. They soften in about the same amount of time the broth from the boiling chicken is done. I pour the broth through a strainer, to separate the liquid from the bones and skin. And add the broth to the pot with the vegetables.*

*It's a very earthy soup. Carrots and onions are roots, and hence move the qi downward in the body, helping promote the digestive process. Celery is a stalk, sprouting upward, so it moves the body's energy up, directing the healing to the lungs and head (sinus, nose, ears, throat). Onions are hot and spicy, moving energy up and out to the body's surface.*

*Adding the chopped-up chicken meat further supports flavor and increases the qi of the broth. I like adding Herbs De Provence in chicken soup, along with salt and pepper. This blend of herbs is considered "woody." The herbs are green and leafy, part of the wood element, which supports the digestive energy, particularly the liver and gallbladder energy, helping us with detoxification. The lavender in the herb blend also helps the energy rise up to the head and lungs, supporting the immune system even more. Salt brings out the flavor of the chicken. Without enough salt, the soup may not have enough flavor, too much salt and you lose the flavor to the salt. But it takes more than you think to adequately season the chicken soup!*

*I like to add some peas to the pot, frozen will do in the wintertime. If need be, feel free to add a box of chicken stock to the broth.*

*In about 45 minutes, your kitchen will be transformed into a cozy, nourishing, yummy place with homemade chicken soup! If you'd like, add rice to the soup for more interest. Rice also brings the grain to the soup to further enhance the earth element's nourishment and makes this a complete meal. Add a little Parsley - it soothes the heart.*

## INGREDIENTS

1 deli chicken, cooked, meat removed from the bones and set in a bowl. (Put the bones and skin in a pot on the stove and cover the carcass with water. Boil for 30-45 minutes to make chicken broth for the soup.)
1 tbsp. olive oil
2 onions, chopped
2 carrots, chopped
2 celery stalks, chopped
1 tsp. thyme or Herbs de Provence
2 tsp. salt

## DIRECTIONS

Heat 1 tbsp. olive oil in a big soup pot.
Add the chopped vegetables and saute until soft.
Add the herbs and 2 tsp. salt.
After the chicken bones and skin are cooked (you will know when they are done because the odor will be released from the bones), strain the broth from the skin and bones.
Add the broth to the pot of vegetables. You may supplement more broth from boxed chicken broth if your homemade broth is too weak. I like the Pacific brand of organic chicken broth. Finally, add the chopped chicken meat to the pot.
Bring to a boil, then reduce heat to a simmer for 20 minutes.
Taste and add salt if the flavor seems wimpy.

*Note: Chicken requires a lot more salt than you'd think in order to be tasty.*

Variations:
Add 1 c. cooked rice to the pot.
Add 1 c. frozen or fresh peas to the pot.

CHINESE MEDICINE REFERENCES

**Chicken** — Meats are warming, in general. "Meat" is the muscle of the animal. When we eat muscle, we nourish our muscles. In the case of poultry, red meat comes from the muscles used in flying and running. They're red because these muscles (wings and legs/thighs) require more red blood in order to move. "White meat" refers to the muscles that are not used for movement, such as the breast. There is less blood flow to these muscles, so they don't turn red. Chicken comes from the earth levels of our food model. It has energy to nourish the stomach, pancreas, spleen.

# Sausage & Bean Soup

### Serves 4-6 | Cook time: 1 hour

*This is an easy, quick soup to make and it is one of my kids' favorites. Combining beans and sausage means there's a lot of protein packed into this soup.*

## INGREDIENTS

1 lb. mild or spicy Italian sausage roll
2 medium onions, chopped
2 carrots, chopped
2 celery stalks, chopped
3 oz. prosciutto, chopped
1 tsp. Herbs de Provence
4 c. chicken broth
2 cans of white beans, Great Northern or Cannellini (don't drain)

## DIRECTIONS

Cook the sausage in a skillet over medium heat.

While the sausage is browning, heat 1 tbsp. olive oil in a large pot (I prefer a Dutch oven) and add the onions, carrots, and celery to cook until they soften.

Next, add the prosciutto and the Herbs de Provence.

When the sausage is done cooking, allow it to cool a little, and then slice it into 1-inch thick pieces.

Add the sausage and broth to the big pot.

Finally, add the beans and their juices from the cans.

Heat until gently boiling, then reduce heat to simmer for 10 minutes.

Turn off the heat and allow the soup to cool for 15 minutes more to marry the flavors.

Bring it back to simmer before serving.

---

CHINESE MEDICINE REFERENCES

The basis for most soups and many other dishes in Western recipes is carrots, celery, and onion. This is an interesting combination for food energy analysis.

**Carrots** — These root vegetables grow downwards, therefore, they direct energy down in the body. Notice how old carrots grow whiskers? They contain so much energy that even after they are picked, they continue to "grow." That means there is a lot of energy in carrots.

**Celery** — This is a stalk that grows upward, so it directs energy upward in the body. Celery contains a lot of water, it is "yin" in nature and cooling. Notice when you eat celery you feel moisture and coolness in your mouth? Celery directs the qi up to the head, but then it descends back downward, it doesn't have the yang to strongly move up and stay up. (Because it ascends and then descends, it could be good for helping headaches that are hot in nature--templar headaches or high blood pressure headaches, for example).

**Onions** — They are spicy and hot, and they bring the energy upward in the body. Notice when you smell onions how your eyes water and burn? That is the experience of the ascending energy of onions, and the heat in them. Onions are a Wei level food.

These three vegetable "friends" perfectly balance each other energetically. No wonder they get along so well in cooking!

# Split-Pea Soup (vegetarian/vegan)

**Serves 6-8 | Cook time: 1.5 hours**

*This is a simple, old-fashioned pea soup. So satisfying, nothing fancy. My family loves this soup, especially on a cold, Colorado day!*

## INGREDIENTS

1 lb. dried green split peas
3 stalks celery, chopped
3 medium carrots, chopped
1 large yellow onion, chopped
2 c. light vegetable broth

Spices:
1 bay leaf
1 tsp. dried thyme
1 – 1 ½ tsp. sea salt, plus more to taste if you like
smoked paprika, to taste
fresh ground black pepper, to taste

## DIRECTIONS

Rinse the split peas

Combine peas in a large pot with 8 cups of water and the chopped celery, carrots, onion, bay leaf, thyme, and a pinch of smoked paprika.

Bring the water to a boil and cook for about 20 minutes.

Reduce the heat, add 1 tsp. of salt and vegetable broth.

Simmer for about 45 minutes, peas should be soft and tender.

Remove the bay leaf, adjust salt to taste, and add ground pepper to taste.

Add a little more vegetable broth if the soup seems too thick.

Now puree the soup in the blender, little by little, or use an immersion blender (a beloved device for frequent soup cooks!). Some people prefer a rough texture, some a smoother texture — blend to your preference.

Taste again and adjust the salt and pepper as needed.

CHINESE MEDICINE REFERENCES

**Legumes** — Legumes, in general, are an excellent source of protein! Within the legume family, peas are among the easiest to digest, and direct qi downwards.

**Fluids** — Soups nourish stomach yin.

**Peas** — Peas are a springtime vegetable, and belong to the wood element. That means they nourish the liver and gallbladder, which assist in digestion and detox. The liver plays a big role in the immune system because of its detoxifying, or purifying, ability.

**Spices** — If you make it more spicy with the paprika, you increase the warmth of the soup, stimulating heat production in your body. If you feel chilled, this can be very helpful for healing. If you tend to run warm anyway, consider using less or no paprika, to allow your body to balance its internal temperature and nourish the yin fluids as much as possible. Too much heat production in your body dries out the body fluids, which negatively impacts your immune system.

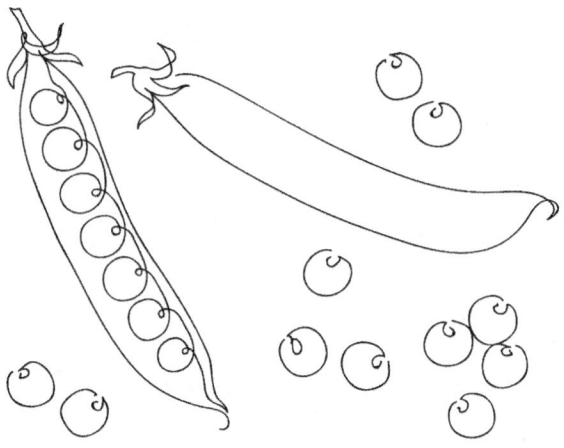

# Cottage Pie

**4-6 servings**
Cook time: around 1 hour 10 minutes if you are making mashed potatoes.
It's around 50 minutes if you are using leftover mashed potatoes.

---

*This recipe has two parts. I like to make it when there are leftover mashed potatoes.*
*Of course, you may make the mashed potatoes just for this dish, too.*

## MASHED POTATOES

### INGREDIENTS

2 lbs. potatoes peeled (unless you use red potatoes or Yukon Gold – their skins are edible)
1 c. milk or chicken broth
salt and pepper

Optional:
2 tbsp. butter

### DIRECTIONS

Boil the potatoes. When they are soft and a knife easily pierces them, take them off the
   stove and drain the water from the pot.
Mash the potatoes with the milk or chicken broth, and add salt and pepper (also add the
   butter at this point, if you choose to include it).
You now have the topping for the cottage pie!

## "PIE"

Preheat oven to 400° F.

### INGREDIENTS

1 lb. ground beef
5-6 green onions (scallions), chopped
2 carrots, grated
1 tsp. of herbs – either thyme, basil, or oregano (or use all 3 herbs, totaling 1 tsp.)
1 tbsp. tomato puree
1 tbsp. Worcester sauce
1 c. beef broth, or bone broth

Optional:
1 c. peas

## DIRECTIONS

Sauté the onions and carrot in a little oil for a few minutes, until they begin to soften.

Add the ground beef, cook for about 20-30 minutes.

Add herbs, tomato puree, Worcester sauce, beef stock (and peas, if using).

Simmer a few minutes and adjust the seasoning.

Using a large oven proof casserole pot (I like to use a Dutch oven), pour in the beef mixture.

Spread the mashed potatoes on top.

You may add a few chopped scallions to the mashed potatoes, if you like.

Put into a preheated oven at 400° F for about 25 minutes.

---

CHINESE MEDICINE REFERENCES

**Meat** — Beef is a warming, Ying level meat. Ground beef can incorporate herbs that aid in digestion.

**Vegetables** — Potatoes are round and grow below ground in the earth, they bring the qi to the center, the stomach. Carrots are a downward-growing root. They direct energy downward in the body, making them good for treating constipation. Green onion is mildly warming, and moves qi downward.

**Spices** — The spices in "this recipe are"woody" and warming -- bay leaf, thyme, basil, and oregano are green, leafy herbs. They all bring energy to lighten the heaviness of the potato by directing qi downwards.

**Peas** — Peas are "optional" because traditionally they are only available in the springtime. But we may get frozen peas, and they add freshness. Peas are also a wood element influence, creating balance This is a lovely dish for cool weather.

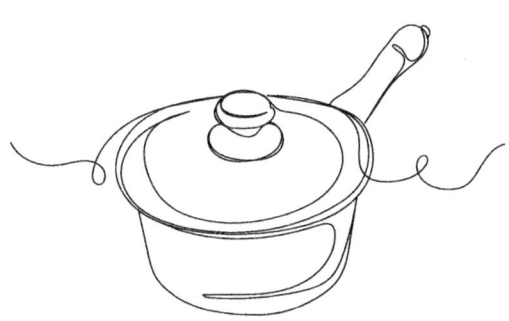

# Greek Lemon Artichoke Chicken

**Serves 6-8 | Prep time: 15 minutes | Cook time: 1 hour**

*This is an adaptation of a recipe from my dear friend's Greek Orthodox Church's cookbook. It's a family favorite, and super easy to make for a dinner party. You may use chicken breasts, or thighs, or a whole chicken cut-up — your choice!*

*I recently served this dish for our annual neighborhood progressive dinner party. There were 10 friends around the table, and everyone loved the meal. One neighbor commented on how well he felt after eating, saying that the meal was not too rich or filling. He felt like he was in good shape to make it to the next house for dessert!*

## INGREDIENTS

8 boneless chicken breasts or 8-10 chicken thighs (bone-in or boneless)
  or a whole chicken, cut into pieces
juice of 1 large lemon
¼ c. olive oil
4-6 cloves garlic, crushed
2 tsp. oregano
1 16 oz. bag of frozen artichoke hearts
1 ½ tsp. salt
1-2 tbsp. butter (optional)

## DIRECTIONS

Preheat oven to 375° F.
Combine oil, lemon juice, garlic, oregano, and salt together and beat with a fork until
  blended to make the marinade.
Dip chicken in marinade and arrange it in a baking dish.
Dot the tops of the chicken with a little butter, if you choose.
Pour the remaining marinade over the chicken and add the frozen artichoke hearts on top.
Bake uncovered for 1 hour.

*Note: I like to serve this with rice and cooked fresh green beans for a complete and energetically balanced meal.*

**Chicken** — Chicken belongs to both the Ying nutritive level, which focuses on the digestive process. Chicken is less warming than red meat.

**Rice** — Rice belongs to the earth element. It aids the stomach by generating fluids, thus making the meat easier to digest.

**Green Beans & Artichokes** — Green beans belong to the wood element -- and they help clear out any stagnant food or qi in the stomach, descending qi.. Artichoke hearts are slightly sour and promote the appetite. "True appetizers" are foods that prepare the stomach and digestive system to receive food by moving qi, releasing any stagnation. This means foods with a sour flavor. Releasing stagnation means relaxing the liver, and so freeing the qi for promoting conversation! When the liver energy is free and relaxed, people are more emotionally relaxed and can connect with each other more easily.

**Marinade** — The lemon and olive oil marinade stimulates the liver and gallbladder to contribute enzymes to help the stomach and small intestine break down the food. Lemon opens to the lung and liver, it's sour and slightly sweet and cooling. It is considered an astringent, and so helps the liver to gather blood, and promotes the appetite. Olive oil is considered bitter and affiliated with the heart and liver. Olives are a fruit, and a true appetizer food, olives promote appetite and digestion. Foods that are related with the heart help it to relax, inviting us to calm down, de-stress, and enjoy one another and express what is in our hearts. Good food truly promotes good digestion and good conversation!

**Note** — This marinade itself is a staple! It can go on meat of any kind. Potatoes roasted in it are divine, and it is good on salads, too. It is a true appetizer, aiding digestion.

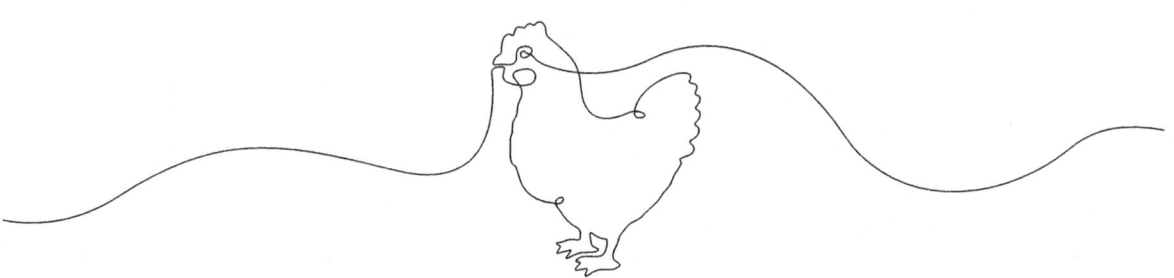

# Spatchcocked Chicken

Serves 6 | Prep time: 30 minutes | Cook time: 1 hour

*This is a simple, tasty way to roast a whole chicken. It is practical and frugal home cooking. Spatchcocking the chicken leads to more even cooking times for breasts and thighs. This means less chance of over-cooking and drying out the breast meat while waiting for the thighs to get done. I've also included a recipe for Chicken Stock that can be made from the leftovers of the Spatchcocked Chicken. This is also an excellent way to roast turkey.*

## INGREDIENTS

1 whole chicken
salt (for the cavity)
salt & pepper to taste
olive oil
herbs/lemon juice

## FOR CHICKEN STOCK

1-2 tsp. salt
2 carrots
1 stalk of celery
pinch of cayenne
a couple ounces of white wine (optional)

## DIRECTIONS

Preheat oven to 425° F.
With kitchen shears, cut through the back of a whole chicken from the vent to neck
   opening, alongside the spine.
Then make a cut through the wide end of the breastbone.
Trim off the tail and wing-tip joints.
Open the bird, clean out the kidneys, wash off the inside.
Then pat dry and salt the inside.
Place the splayed bird with both breasts and legs facing up on a roasting pan (no lid).
Rub with olive oil and season as you wish. For example, use fresh or dried herbs, lemon
   juice, salt, pepper, etc.
Add 4-6 ounces of liquid to the bottom of the pan (white wine works well).
Roast at 425° F for 25 minutes, then reduce heat to 375° F for another 30 minutes.

Check the chicken's internal temperature at this point in the breasts and thighs — aiming for 165-185° F.

When cooked, remove from the oven and let rest for 15 minutes.

Then carve and serve. Save the pan drippings and fat for making chicken stock from the bones.

## CHICKEN STOCK DIRECTIONS

Place the bones of the chicken along with the fat and pan drippings into a stockpot with plenty of water to cover the carcass. (maybe about a gallon or less, depending on the size of the chicken).

Add 1-2 tsp. salt, 2 carrots, 1 stalk of celery.

Add just a pinch of a warming spice, such as cayenne.

Adding a couple ounces of white wine is nice, too, but not essential.

Bring to a boil, then reduce heat to a simmer for 2-3 hours; allow to cool.

Strain and decant into dated freezer containers. Or use the hot stock for soup!

---

CHINESE MEDICINE REFERENCES

**Chicken** — Chicken can be classified as a Ying level food. It nourishes the stomach and digestive tract.

**Turkey** — Turkey is a Wei level meat and relaxes the heart.

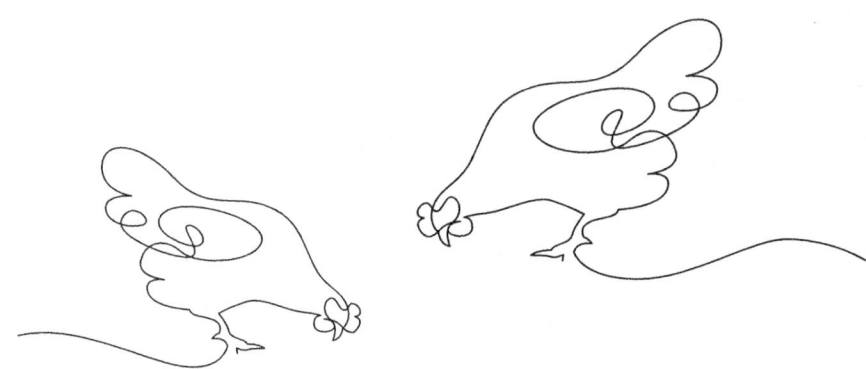

# Smoky Lentil Stew

Serves 4-6   |   Cook time: 1 hour

Lentils are such a friendly food! They are very small beans, and as legumes they deliver protein. They nourish yin in the body. This means that they are cooling and moistening for the stomach and bring this quality energy to the kidneys — very helpful for balancing hormones and strengthening bones. Animal protein is warm and can produce "dampness" if it is fatty. Of course, the stomach needs to be warm in order to digest foods (stomach acid is HOT!), but too much heat causes big problems. We are grateful to legumes in general, and lentils in particular, for giving us protein in a cooling, yin nourishing package. This is important for those who eat mostly meat which makes the stomach too "hot!"

## INGREDIENTS

1 ½ c. lentils
7 c. vegetable or chicken stock
1 c. diced green onion
3 cloves minced garlic
1 c. diced carrot
1 bunch kale, chopped
juice of 1 lemon

Spices
1 tsp. smoked paprika
1 tsp. cumin
salt and pepper to taste

## DIRECTIONS

Heat 1 tbsp. olive oil or coconut oil in a Dutch oven over medium heat.
Add onion and carrot, stir occasionally until tender, about 5 minutes.
Add garlic, smoked paprika, cumin, salt and pepper, cook 1 minute.
Add the lentils, kale, and the stock.
Increase heat to a boil, then reduce heat and simmer until lentils are tender, about 25 minutes.
Add lemon juice, tasting as you go (the amount of lemon may vary with each soup!)
Add kale and simmer longer, until the kale turns bright green.
Serve with a bowl of rice. YUM!

**Lentils** — They are so quick and easy to cook with! Coming from the legume family, they contain the wood element (think helpful for the liver and gallbladder). Lentils are small beans and they "drain damp" from the stomach. That means they help with bloating, indigestion, candida, and inflammation -- all signs of internal "dampness." The color of the lentil shows the element within the wood that it supports. You can use green, red, yellow, white, or brown lentils for this stew.

**Kale** — This leafy green has strong descending energy. Kale nourishes and relaxes the liver.

**Spices** — Smoky paprika, garlic, and onions add heat and lightness to lift the qi in this dish for balance. Do you feel the heat in your mouth and how it lifts up qi in your body when you taste it?

**Boiling** — Cooking via boiling adds water, or yin, to the body. This is so important for stomach health and for the immune system.

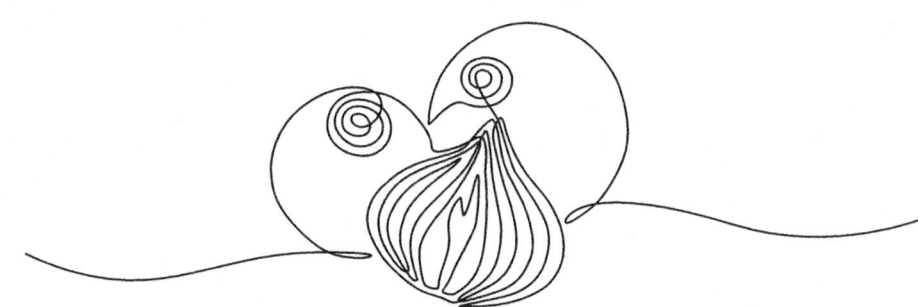

# Manx Lamb Stew

Serves 4-6
Cook time: 1-2 hours; but really, stews taste better the longer they have to simmer,
just watch the liquid — don't let it dry out!

*My mother hails from a small island in the Irish Sea called The Isle of Man. Named for the Celtic Sea deity, Mananan, the Isle of Man is home to a few unusual things. One of my favorites is the four-horned Loaghtan sheep, which my family raised on the farm. The other is Manx cats, tailless cats that have long hind legs, a double coat of fur, big ears and are very affectionate. Growing up I had a Manx cat called Cushag, named after the Isle of Man's national wildflower. This stew is a tribute to Mom and the Loaghtan sheep of her childhood.*

## INGREDIENTS

2-3 lbs. lamb shank. If a shank is not available, try using a bone-in cut of lamb — leg or shoulder cut. It's the bone that gives the best flavor for the stew. Cut the meat off of the bone and slice into bite-size cubes.
1 large onion, diced small
6 potatoes, cut into bite-sized cubes
2 carrots, sliced
1 tbsp. Worcester sauce
1 bay leaf

Optional (and very nice to add):
1 c. peas
2 celery tops with leaves, sliced
parsley, chopped

## DIRECTIONS

In a large pot, cover the lamb bones and the cut-up meat with water (maybe about 6-8 cups of water).
Add the bay leaf and salt and pepper (about 2 tsp. salt and 1 tsp. pepper).
Bring to a boil.
Then turn down the temperature and allow the bone and meat to simmer for about 2 hours. The water will steam off and the broth will become more concentrated and golden-colored, it will smell delicious.
Simmer until broth is reduced to about 4 c.

Take the stew off the heat and allow to cool. Then you can scrape the fat off the top of the broth and discard it.

Add onion, potatoes, carrots, and Worcester sauce and simmer until vegetables are soft (maybe around 30 minutes).

If adding peas, put them in at the end and get them warmed into the stew before serving it.

If adding celery, toss it into the pot along with the carrots, onions, and potatoes to boil.

Some folks like a little parsley on top of the stew when they serve it.

---

CHINESE MEDICINE REFERENCES

**Lamb** —Lamb is a very warming meat. It is very nice for warming the blood in the cold wintertime.

**Vegetables** —Onion, carrot, and celery (the three vegetable friends) are a balanced combination of energy for the stew. They distribute energy throughout the digestive system and body.

**Potatoes** —Potatoes are tubers, they gather qi in the center of our body (in the stomach). They are cooling and support the stomach, spleen, and pancreas. They don't move qi, the other foods in the recipe need to do this in order to digest easily.

# Bean & Vegetable Chili

Serves 4-6
Cook time: 1 hour (If using raw beans, allow for soaking overnight)

*Ok, I admit: I often use canned beans for chili. \*gasp!\* It's sad because taking the time to cook dried beans is not that much trouble, it's less expensive — and, it's more tasty. The reason I often fail at this is due to a lack of organization! When I need a quick, filling, and crowd-pleasing dinner, I can easily throw this chili together (using canned beans) and call it good. I'll give you the recipe both ways — using dried beans and using canned beans. Chances are, you are better organized than I am, and can make the dried bean recipe. Try it! Naturally, everyone has their own opinion of how spicy chili should be. Feel free to add or subtract the amount of oregano, cumin, or chili powder as you prefer. For that matter, feel free to add or subtract the vegetables as you prefer. This is a forgiving recipe. The idea is to allow the beans, vegetables, and spices to blend flavors as they simmer. This part takes a little time.*

*This is a meal in a bowl. It's nice to serve with avocado slices, fresh cilantro leaves, lime wedges, and shredded cheddar cheese. My family likes cornbread with this chili, too.*


## DRIED BEANS

### INGREDIENTS

1 c. dried red kidney beans
1 c. dried pinto beans
1 c. dried garbanzo beans


### DIRECTIONS

Wash the beans separately.
You may cook your beans together if you know they are relatively fresh; if not, then cook
  them separately because garbanzos tend to take longer to cook than kidneys or pintos.
Use 4 c. water per 1 c. of beans.
Put the beans in the water, bring to a boil, and simmer for about an hour.

*Note: The older the beans, the longer the cooking time needed — maybe 20-30 minutes longer. The beans should be tender to bite, but not mushy, when cooked. Add ¾ tsp. salt once they are cooked, and simmer for 5 minutes more, then turn off the heat. (If you add salt too early, the beans will stay hard.) Now, these are ready to add to your chili.*

If you are using canned beans:
1 can red kidney beans
1 can pinto beans
1 can garbanzo beans

Simply drain the cans of any liquid.

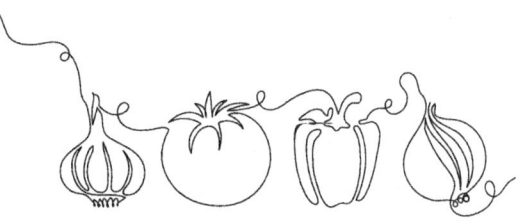

## VEGETABLES

6-8 green onions, chopped
2 cloves of garlic, chopped
2 carrots, diced
1 bell pepper, cored and diced
1 bunch green chard, chopped leaves only
½ c. cilantro, chopped
1 28-oz. can fire-roasted chopped tomatoes
3 tbsp. olive oil
dash of sea salt
1 tbsp. dried oregano
1 tbsp. ground cumin
2 ½ tbsp. chili powder

## DIRECTIONS

In a large pan, sauté onions in olive oil until they soften.
Add garlic, and a pinch of salt.
Cook at medium heat.
Add diced carrots and bell peppers and sauté 10 minutes more.
Add the spices: cumin, oregano, and chili powder to the vegetables and stir for 1 minute.
Add the tomatoes, beans, and liquid. NOTE: If you are using canned beans, add 2 cans of
    water.
After about 30 minutes of cooking, add the chopped chard and cilantro, and taste for salt.
Simmer for 30 minutes more. Check to make sure it does not get dry, if so, add more water.

CHINESE MEDICINE REFERENCES

*Legumes (beans)* — Another meal made of legumes, the wonderful protein source from vegetables! Beans belong to the wood element and move downwardly to assist digestion.

*Vegetables & Spices* — Most of the vegetables in this chili are neutral and descending qi. The spices are warming..

Together, the legumes and the vegetable/spice mixture create a complementary balance of energy moving upward (warming spices) and downward (beans).

*NOTE: The more spicy you make your chili, the more you are stimulating the heating and drying in the body. On the flip side, the more liquid and less spicy you make it, the more you are contributing to the stomach yin fluids that aid the immune system and digestive health. The choice is yours! If you tend to eat more meat, it's good to enjoy the more "cooling" benefits of legumes to balance the "heat" of meat in your typical diet. If you tend to eat a more vegetarian diet, you will need more "heat" from spices in order to support your stomach which needs a hot environment in order to digest well.*

# Braised Chard with Garlic

Serves 4  |  **Prep time:** 10 minutes  |  **Cook time:** 15 minutes

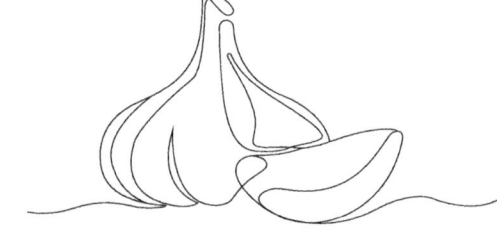

## INGREDIENTS

1 bunch of chard
1 or 2 cloves of garlic
1 tbsp. olive oil
1 tsp. salt
1 tbsp. butter

## DIRECTIONS

Wash and cut the chard into 1-inch slices, including the stems. Peel a clove or two of garlic, and slice it into small pieces.

Put 1 tbsp. olive oil in a pan, add the chard stems.

Sauté the stems for about 5 minutes, until they are softening, then add the leaves and 1 tbsp. of water to the pan.

Put the sliced garlic on top of the leaves, sprinkle about 1 tsp. of salt over the top.

I like to add about 1 tbsp. butter, cut into little chunks, tucked into the leaves.

Then put a tightly fitted lid over the pan and braise on medium heat for 8-10 minutes, until the leaves are wilted.

**Chard** — Chard is a liver food. The liver is the organ of detoxification. It is also associated with the smooth flow of our emotions. This yummy green leafy vegetable is so good at relaxing the liver, which means relaxing emotions, too. Chard also nourishes the blood as it cools and detoxifies it. Chard's green color is the signature of the wood element. Its leaves grow up and open, bringing openness or relaxation to the liver. The message of this plant is "relax and chill." It guides the qi and blood downward, so it is helpful to regulate high blood pressure and it's good for treating PMS and migraines.

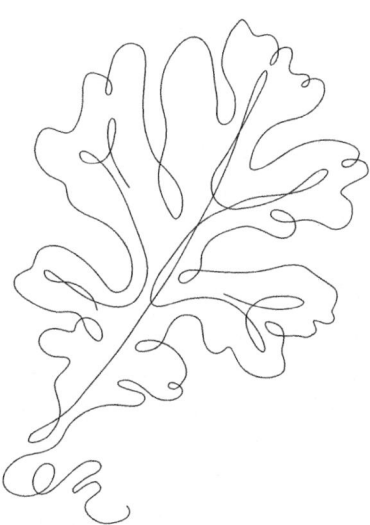

# Eiko's Sesame Spinach

Serves 4-6    |    Cook time: 20 minutes

I lived in Japan for 2 years during the early part of my education in Traditional East Asian Medicine. As it goes when we are open to energy and guidance from the mystical qi, I met some amazing people who helped to shape my experience of living and learning, and we became friends. One of those friends materialized in the form of weekly Japanese cooking classes in her kitchen! She mentored me through the grocery store (I couldn't read any labels, nor recognize many foods), and into the kitchen. There were so many shapes and sizes of knives! Plus, she shared the sacred ways of rice with me — who knew? And then there were the dining table manners: It's not just about chopsticks! It was pure heaven! Eiko Fujii was her name, and she was one of the blessings of support and nourishment during my student days in Japan. We worked our way around her tiny kitchen, and she taught me her wisdom of life via cooking. This recipe is one of the results of her instruction. Thank you, Eiko!

## INGREDIENTS

2 bunches of fresh spinach, about ¾ lb.
2 tbsp. black or white sesame seeds
2 tsp. sesame oil
2 tsp. tamari
2 tsp. mirin

## DIRECTIONS

Boil some water in a saucepan.
While water is heating, thoroughly wash the spinach.
Gently put the spinach in the boiling water for only 1-2 minutes to blanch the leaves — making sure it's less than 3 minutes.
Remove the spinach from the water, run the leaves under cold water and then squeeze out any remaining water. Get it as dry as possible.
Lay the spinach down neatly on a chopping block with all of the ends together (making the leaves together, too). Cut it into inch-wide strips.
Set into a serving bowl.
Stir the sesame seeds in a medium-hot fry pan until they are dry.
Combine the sesame oil, tamari, and mirin in a small bowl and whisk together.
Pour over the spinach.
Sprinkle the sesame oil and sesame seeds over the spinach and serve.

**Spinach** — Spinach is the wood element — leafy, green food. It is energetically cold, bitter, sweet, and descending. This makes it a good diuretic as it clears built-up fluids, opens the lungs, and relaxes the liver. It is good to eat it in rotation with other greens, and not too often. Because spinach is cold and bitter in nature, it is best to eat it wilted or blanched. Steaming bitter vegetables actually increases their bitterness. And eating spinach raw only increases its coldness. So, wilting it is best — just warm it until the leaves soften and gently collapse.

**Sesame seeds** — Sesame seeds, and all seeds, are classified as kidney energy foods. Seeds contain the beginning of life, so they nourish the foundation of life — kidney energy and the Yuan level of foods.

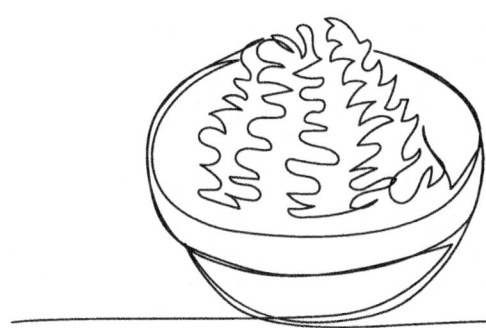

# Roasted Broccoli

**Serves 4-6** | **Cook time: 25 minutes**

## INGREDIENTS

½ onion
1 tsp. fresh rosemary leaves
1 lemon, quartered
1 head of broccoli
1 tbsp. olive oil
salt & pepper to taste

## DIRECTIONS

Preheat oven to 450° F.
Mince ½ onion.
Finely chop 1 tsp. fresh rosemary leaves.
Cut a lemon into quarters.
Wash broccoli and cut the florets apart. Cut up the stem into bite sizes chunks.
Line a baking sheet with foil (for easy clean-up).
Drizzle 1 tbsp. olive oil on the foil-covered sheet and toss the broccoli and onion with salt and pepper to taste.
Roast on the middle rack for 12-15 minutes until browned and tender.
When you take them out of the oven, squeeze lemon juice on top and toss them together.

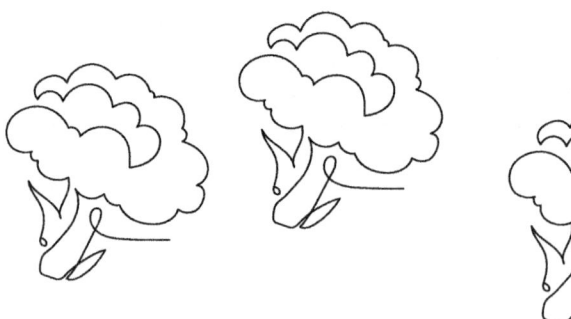

**Broccoli** — Think about the way that broccoli grows. It has little florets in bunches, and they circle around each other forming a spherical bouquet. That circular growth pattern is the signature of the earth element family of food. Broccoli is that beautiful color of green, which is the signature of the wood element. Therefore, when we eat broccoli, we are nourishing the stomach, spleen, and pancreas system (earth element), as well as the liver and gallbladder system (wood element).

**Roasting** — Roasting food in the oven, without a lid, is a cooking method that puts heat into the food, condenses the food, and dries it. This is the signature of the water element (kidney energy). It consolidates the qi in the food and makes it concentrated.

**Medicine of the Dish** — Putting all of this together, roasted broccoli nourishes the stomach, liver, and kidney systems. From the Western nutrition point of view, broccoli has calcium (kidney energy) and aids in digestion (stomach and liver energy).

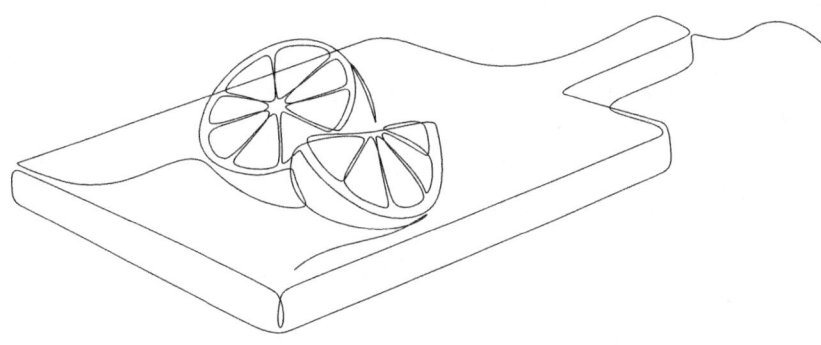

# Roasted Brussels Sprouts

Serves 4-6   |   Cook time: 30 minutes

*I became a Brussels sprout convert after a friend told me her children LOVE Brussels sprouts. I couldn't believe it! I was raised with the occasional steamed Brussels sprouts, which were bitter, and thus, very occasional. She told me to roast them in the oven. I tried, and my children loved them, too!*

## INGREDIENTS

1.5 lbs. Brussels sprouts
3-5 tbsp. olive oil
2-3 pinches sea salt
parchment paper

## DIRECTIONS

Preheat oven to 400° F.
Rinse the Brussels sprouts.
Peel off any unfresh (old and wilted) leaves, and trim the bottoms.
Cut in half, lengthwise. My husband likes to cut out the core of the sprout, but I usually leave them, just make a slit into the core so it can soften as it cooks.
In a bowl, toss the sprouts with olive oil and salt — enough of each to lightly coat all the sprouts.
Place the sprouts on a cooking sheet covered with parchment paper. Spread them apart, so they are not covering each other. They need their space to cook evenly.
Roast for around 25 minutes*, turning them over once or twice while they are roasting. When they're done, they should be tender enough for a fork to pierce them (but not mushy) and a little brown.

*Note: Cooking times will vary depending on the size of the sprouts and their density, the way you cut them and handle their core, and when you turn them — and of course, your oven. If they are small, cooking may be done in just 12-15 minutes! So, pay attention to them, they will let you know when they are ready.*

**Brussels sprouts** — These veggies grow in little spirals of leaves, curling inwardly while they grow up on stalks. They are a member of the cabbage family, their siblings include broccoli, cauliflower, collards, kale, and cabbage. They nourish the stomach, spleen, liver and gall bladder. They are slightly warming, but also clear damp heat and moisten the intestines. Other vegetables are delicious when prepared and roasted the same way. Try broccoli, beets, carrots, parsnips, winter squashes, and sweet potatoes.

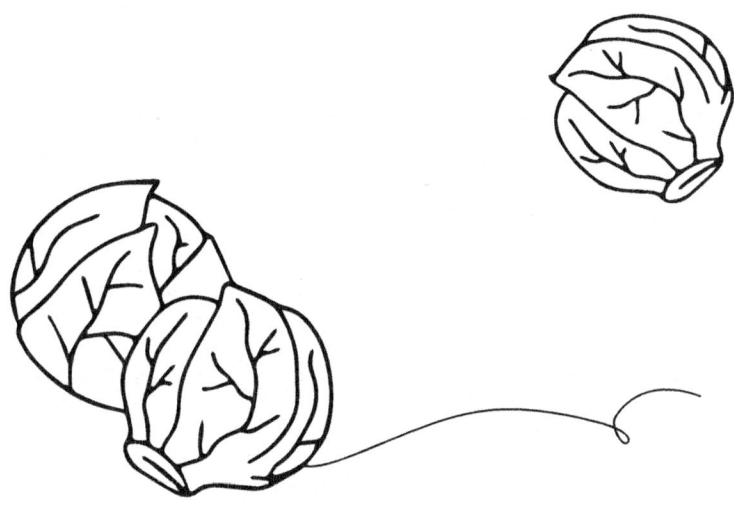

# Roasted Chard or Kale with Feta

Serves 4-6  |  Cook time: 50 minutes

*This is another quick-cooking and crowd-pleasing vegetable recipe from the wood element, relaxing and strengthening the liver. Even my Dad, who doesn't like green vegetables (especially kale), loves this! Sweet potato leaves are also delicious when cooked this way. If you are lucky enough to grow them in your garden, try some like this!*

## INGREDIENTS

1 bunch of chard or kale or a mixture
½ an onion, finely diced
2-3 tbsps. olive oil (1 tbsp. for baking sheet, 1-2 tbsp. drizzled on top)
pinch of salt
½ c. feta cheese
1 tsp. fresh-squeezed lemon juice (optional)

## DIRECTIONS

Preheat oven to 350° F.
Wash a bunch of chard or kale or both together.
Cut the leaves in one-inch slices. NOTE: Kale leaves may be peeled away from the thick
  stalks, only use their leaves. Chard stalks are softer and delicious, cut ½-inch thick.
Cut up ½ of an onion, into a fine dice.
Line a baking sheet with foil.
Pour 1 tbsp. olive oil on the sheet, toss the chard stems and onion onto the sheet, and
  roast for about 15 minutes, until soft and beginning to brown.
Take the sheet out of the oven, add the leaves and drizzle 1-2 tbsp. olive oil on top and mix
  together to coat the leaves, using tongs.
Sprinkle a pinch of salt and ½ c. feta cheese on top. Roast in the oven for 20 minutes.

Optional: If you'd like, when you remove the pan from the oven, squeeze 1 tsp. fresh lemon
juice over the top, and serve.

**Kale and Chard** — Both of these are broad leaf, green vegetables. This type of leafy vegetable unfurls its leaves as it grows upward, stretching up and out to the world. When the liver energy is smoothly flowing and the heart is nourished, we, too, feel open-hearted and freely flowing in our lives. Eating this food encourages the body to follow the signature of the energy and open and flow, relaxing and nourishing the blood. Kale is course, and has a downward moving quality so it helps move stagnation, it also builds blood. Chard is soothing and cooling for the Liver, descending energy.

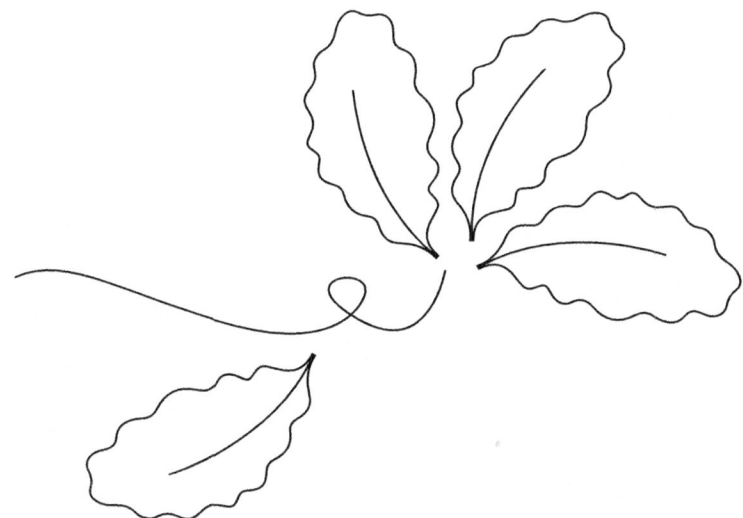

# Stewed Okra

Serves 4-6 | Cook time: 25 minutes

*This is a recipe from my friend, Ellen, who has taught me several wonderful Greek dishes. She owned a Greek restaurant for a while and I benefited in many ways from her cooking wisdom and patience. Thanks, Ellen!*

## INGREDIENTS

1.5 lbs. okra, fresh or frozen
Note: Okra can be difficult to find fresh, so I use frozen okra. If you can find fresh, wash it and carefully trim the pointy end and the end next to the stem — not too close to the pod— and sprinkle vinegar over it, letting it soak in for half an hour.
½ c. olive oil
2 medium onions, sliced
3-4 garlic cloves, sliced
2 c. tomatoes, chopped
2 tbsp. fresh parsley, chopped
1 bay leaf

## DIRECTIONS

In a heavy pot, sauté the onions and garlic in ¼ c. olive oil until the onions turn translucent.
Add salt and pepper to taste.
Add the tomatoes, parsley, bay leaf, and some water (about ¼ c.) so that it is not too dry and simmer. Rinse the okra.
Pour ¼ c. olive oil in a second frying pan
Add okra and sauté for a few minutes.
Remove from the heat.
Add the okra to the sauce and simmer until tender.

---

CHINESE MEDICINE REFERENCES

**Okra** — Okra is slightly slimy, which is the food quality of the small intestine! The small intestine is nourished by food with a slippery quality to it, helping the downward movement of qi.

**Garlic/Onion** — Two of the most heating and dehydrating things we can eat, so eat them carefully and seldomly. Instead, cook and eat green onions with abandon!

**Tomato** — As members of the nightshade family, tomatoes raise heat in the blood and move the blood. However, if they are cooked for more than 3 hours, their energy softens and they can actually clear heat in the blood!

# Steamed Greens

**Serves 4-6** | **Prep. time: 10 minutes**

*The nicest, simplest way to cook green vegetables is to steam them. Here is an example , but you may substitute almost any green vegetable. The only caution is with bitter greens- they get more bitter through steaming, so I like to braise them instead.*

## INGREDIENTS

1 bunch of chard
1 tbsp. olive oil
salt

## DIRECTIONS

Rinse chard and cut into 3 inch strips, including the stems.
Put a pot of water on the stove, with a steamer basket inside. Bring the water to a boil.
   Add the chard. Steam until the leaves wilt, maybe 3-5 minutes.
   Once the steaming is done, remove the chard from the basket and gently put in a bowl.
Lightly pour a little olive oil over it, add a pinch of salt. Toss with tenderness. Wahla!
A simple and quick  and delicious green vegetable for your meal!

---

CHINESE MEDICINE REFERENCES

Vegetables and fruits tend to have strong directionality, they move food downwardly. This facilitates good digestion. Tubers and grains tend to consolidate qi in the center, in the stomach. The health of the spleen/pancreas shows in our ability digest grains and tubers. The spleen can't digest if it gets damp. The spleen can get damp from food sitting in the stomach for too long. This is why eating lots of cooked vegetables with grains or tubers is so important.

# Moroccan Carrots

Serves 4-6  |  Cook time: 10 minutes

*This recipe is a simple way to dress carrots up for a warming, winter, dinner version of their inherent sweetness.*

## INGREDIENTS

3 c. chopped carrots (1-2 inches thick)
1 tsp. ground cinnamon
1 tsp. ground ginger
3 tsp. olive oil
½ c. honey
3 tsp. vinegar
1 tbsp. fresh chopped parsley or cilantro

## DIRECTIONS

Cook the carrots in boiling water for 5 minutes, until tender.
Drain.
Toss carrots with all other ingredients.
Serve warm.

---

CHINESE MEDICINE REFERENCES

**Carrots** — Are root vegetables, and move qi downward.

**Vinegar** — Balances the sweetness of carrots and spices with a warming and astringent quality, aiding digestion.

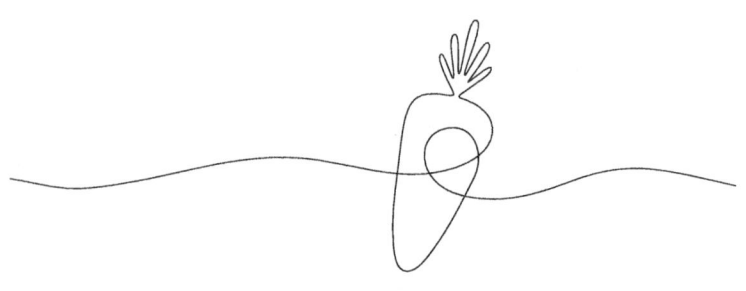

# Roasted Root Vegetables 3 Ways

*Here are several versions of these wonderful fall and winter, roastie-toastie blends of vegetables. These are so easy to make — the peeling is the part that requires the most work. Once that's done, just dress the veggies and slip them into the oven for about 1 hour to transform them into a nutritious and delicious meal component.*

## Roasted Winter Roots

**Each recipe serves 4-6 | Prep time: 20 minutes | Cook time: 1 hour**

### INGREDIENTS

1 ½ lbs. small red potatoes, cut in half
1 bunch of slender carrots
½-¾ lb. pearl onions or sliced yellow onions
2-3 tbsp. olive oil
thyme – 1 tbsp. fresh or 1 tsp. dried
rosemary – 1 tbsp. fresh or 1 tsp. dried

On the stove:
⅓ c. chicken broth
⅓ c. red wine
¼ c. balsamic vinegar

### DIRECTIONS

Mix the veggies in a roasting pan with olive oil and herbs.

Cook at 400° F for about 1 hour, until the vegetables are tender. Then remove from the oven. You may be perfectly happy with the yummy vegetables from the oven as is. But if you need to increase the energetic heat in the vegetables, then the stove top liquids are a nice addition.

On the stove: Heat together chicken broth, red wine, and balsamic vinegar.

Stir the warmed liquids into the browned, sticky vegetables and drippings in the pan.

Serve hot.

# Fancy Roasted Winter Roots

*This is the essence of the pleasure of winter vegetables.*

## INGREDIENTS

1 lb. rutabagas
1 lb. turnips
1 lb. yams
1 lb. fennel
1 lb. carrots
2 lbs. onions

4 tbsp. olive oil
2 tsp. salt
black pepper to taste
2 tsp. fresh thyme or 1 tsp. dried
2 tsp. fresh sage or 1 tsp. dried
3 tbsp. dry sherry

## DIRECTIONS

Preheat oven to 375° F.

Peel and dice all the vegetables into about 1-inch cubes, onions can be larger since they aren't as dense.

Mix the vegetables with olive oil and herbs and sherry salt and pepper. You may season to taste, varying the amounts of herbs; the amounts listed will add subtle flavor and not dominate the vegetables.

Spread the veggies into 2 shallow baking pans (I like to line mine with foil for easy clean-up).

Mix the veggies a few times during roasting and switch the pans between upper and lower oven racks. The veggies will reduce in volume as they cook, when finished there should be about 8 cups of caramelized, browned around the edges, yummy veggies!

Ideas: Put these into a soup, adding vegetable broth and barley. Eat them as is, or roll into a tortilla with scrambled eggs. Add them to greens, or a risotto.

# Roastie-Toastie Potatoes

**Serves 6 | Cook time: 1 hour 10 minutes**

*This is the roastie-toastie potato recipe of my childhood, still simple and still the best! The secret to good roastie-toasties is to boil the potatoes first, then roast them in a hot oven.*

## INGREDIENTS

2 lbs. of baby red potatoes or baby Yukon gold potatoes
3 tbsp. butter

1 tsp. salt
pepper to taste

## DIRECTIONS

Preheat oven to 400° F.
Boil potatoes. If you like them bite-sized, then cut them in half.
When they are softening, transfer the potatoes out of the boiling water and into a roasting pan. Add butter, salt, and pepper to taste.
Roast in the oven until browned, about 30-45 minutes.
Stir the potatoes halfway through cooking time, so they brown on all sides.

Ideas: Of course, you may add peeled and diced yams to the roasting in the oven phase, if you like mixed potatoes. Yams add sweetness to the dish. Yams are a little more difficult to digest when mixed with other foods. You are better off eating them on their own with various toppings.

CHINESE MEDICINE REFERENCES

**Root vegetables** — All vegetables are part of the Ying nutritive level of foods. This means that they fortify the digestive organs (stomach, spleen, pancreas, and small intestine). Roots grow downwardly into the earth. Thus, roots nourish earth organs and move qi downward in the body. This helps with elimination. Adding wine, or sherry, or even butter, turns up the heat element in these recipes, perfect for winter warming.

**Potatoes** — Potatoes are tubers, they nourish and consolidate qi in the stomach.

# Stuffed Spaghetti Squash

**Serves 4-6  |  Cook time: 30-40 minutes**

*For a light summer or early fall dish, this is a winner! This recipe is from my friend, Katie Hardie, who is a nutritional consultant and trainer for athletes. She has shared this and many other simple and delicious recipes for this book. Whenever I make this on a summer day, I think of her and her clear focus and dedication. It inspires a light, clear energy!*

## INGREDIENTS

1 spaghetti squash, cut in half long-ways
1 bunch of spinach, chopped
2 cloves garlic, minced
2 large tomatoes, diced
½ c. kalamata olives, sliced in half
1 ½ tsp. of a combination of basil, oregano, thyme, and rosemary

## DIRECTIONS

Heat oven to 400° F.
Split the squash, remove the seeds from the center, sprinkle with salt and pepper.
Place squash face down on a baking sheet, roast until cooked through and tender when pricked with a knife — so the "noodles" can pull out with a fork.
Meanwhile, sauté the spinach, garlic, and tomatoes in ghee, butter, or olive oil.
Sprinkle with salt and Italian herbs.
Add kalamata olives and then combine with the spaghetti squash.

**Spaghetti Squash** — Squash is the champion for the earth element, stomach and spleen, and pancreas. It supports healing and draining dampness from the stomach and digestive system, aiding the Small Intestine.. Serve this with a little meat or legumes, and a grain, and you have a complete dinner.

**Herbs** — The herbs in this dish (basil, oregano, thyme, and rosemary) are members of the "wood" family. We use their leaves in cooking to contribute flavor (obviously) and also stimulate digestion by giving warmth and descending movement of qi so that the food doesn't sit in the stomach and feel heavy, creating food stagnation.

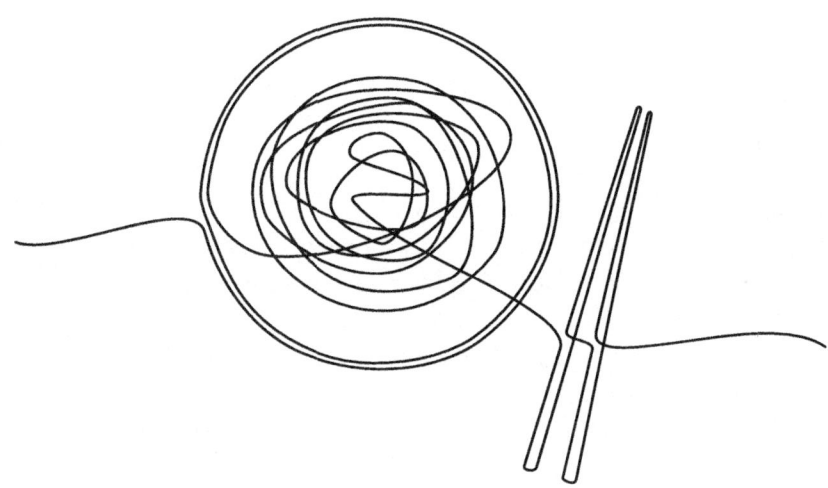

# Roasted Delicata Squash & Sage

**Serves 4** | **Prep time: 10 minutes** | **Cook time: 30-40 minutes**

*This is perhaps my favorite squash and recipe for squash. When autumn squashes come to market, it makes me so happy to find delicata, like seeing an old friend after an absence! Not only is this squash beautiful with its green and yellow stripes, but it is also sweet and delicious, and easy to make. All the best things in one!*

## INGREDIENTS

1 delicata squash, washed and sliced lengthwise, seeds scooped out
¼ c. olive oil
1 tablespoon chopped sage
¼-½ tsp. salt
¼-½ tsp. pepper

## DIRECTIONS

Preheat oven to 400° F.
Pour olive oil into a small bowl
Add sage and muddle with a fork or spoon.
Add the salt and pepper.
Set aside.
Slice the squash lengthwise, so it's in quarters.
Place the slices on a shallow baking sheet. (I line the sheet with foil, for easy cleanup.)
Drizzle the oil infusion over each slice of squash, and massage the oil over the squash so that it's completely coated.
Set the tray in the oven and bake for 30-40 minutes, until the delicata can be easily pierced with a fork through its skin.
Serve immediately and enjoy eating the entire slice, skin and all! YUM!

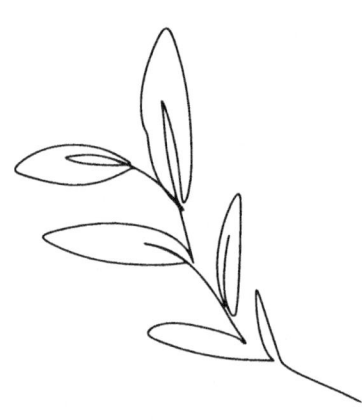

**Squash, and all yellow/orange colored vegetables** —— These are members of the "earth" category of food. This means that they support the stomach and digestion process. They also strengthen the stomach, giving it the *energy it needs in order to digest food.*

A baby is a beginner eater, and we are training a baby's digestive system when we introduce food. It is best for the newly developing digestive system if we begin introducing food only when a baby asks for it by reaching out or grabbing solid food. Then we serve only warm, cooked, pureed food. Cooked, pureed squashes bring moisture, supporting stomach yin.

Squashes, yam, and sweet potato are usually the first solid foods for a baby to eat after mother's milk and rice congee because they nourish the stomach and digestive system. All squash is in this same category of first foods. After a baby has tried many yellow/orange vegetables, then we slowly move on to introduce other colors of food, always returning to the yellow/orange foods in between the new foods so that the stomach may easily receive the new food and grow strong between "introductions."

After vegetables have been intoduced, we bring fruit to the baby. Fruits are cold in nature and therefore not as strengthening for the beginner digestive system of a baby to handle. The last category of food to introduce is protein.

Likewise, if you are suffering from digestive disorders, retraining the digestive system to accept good food begins with the squash family.

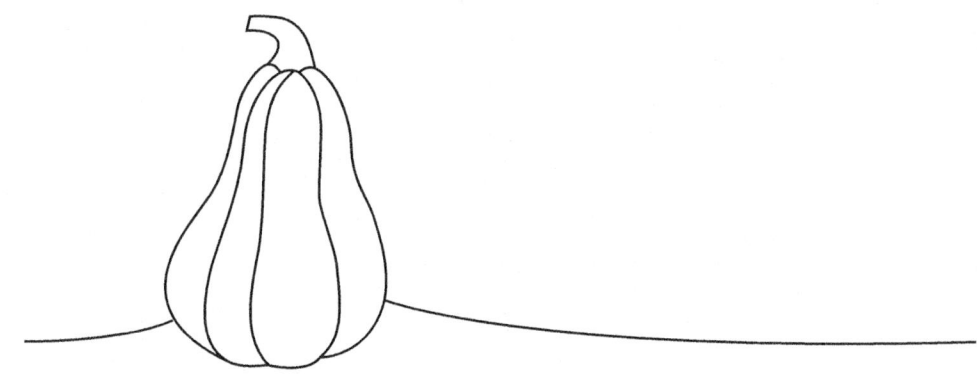

# Sauteed Zucchini

**Serves: 2-4  |  Cook time: 10 minutes**

## INGREDIENTS

1 zucchini, sliced into medallions
1 tbsp. olive oil
salt and pepper to taste

## DIRECTIONS

Pour olive oil into a saute pan, under medium-low heat.
Add the zucchini and salt and pepper.
Allow it to turn light brown.
Then gently turn the medallions over to the other side, and cook — maybe only 1 minute
   longer.

---

**CHINESE MEDICINE REFERENCES**

**Zucchini** — Zucchini is an important food to promote the 6th taste: bland. Bland foods open to the urinary bladder and small intestine. They help the body cleanse. Other bland foods are bland melons, cucumber, and tofu. Cantonese cooking uses a lot of bland foods, and is very tasty. Bland doesn't mean lack of flavor. It means that the food's directionality promotes the healthy function of digestion by cleaning the system.

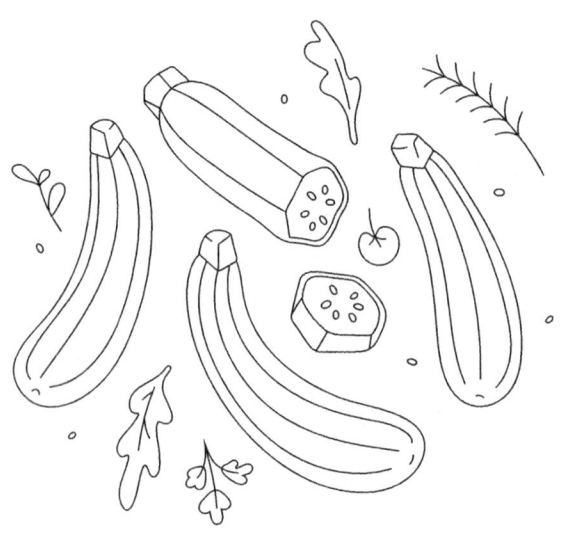

# Barbecued Yellow Squash

**Serves 2-4  |  Cook time: 15 minutes**

INGREDIENTS

1 yellow squash
1 tbsp. olive oil
1 tsp. Herbs de Provence

DIRECTIONS

Get a large rectangle of foil.
Put the olive oil in the center of the foil.
Add the squash over the oil, along with the herbs sprinkled on top and a little salt if you'd like.
Fold the foil over the squash to form a sealed tent.
Place the foil container of squash over the barbecue on medium heat. (If using the oven, cook at 350° F.)
Let the squash cook until it is tender, maybe 10 minutes.
Open the foil tent and serve the squash. Yum!

---

CHINESE MEDICINE REFERENCES

**Yellow squash** — Yellow summer squash is very moist inside, it nourishes stomach yin. It is in the "bland" food category. It is slightly slimy (like zucchini) in a good way! The small intestine thrives on this type of texture in food. It is soothing to the small intestine and urinary bladder, supporting their healthy functions. Barbecued foods infuses fire/heat into the food, and slightly dries food out.

# Baked Butternut Squash

Serves 4-6  |  Prep time: 10 minutes  |  Cook time: 45 minutes

## INGREDIENTS

1 butternut squash, washed
1 tbsp. olive oil
salt and pepper to taste

## DIRECTIONS

Preheat the oven to 350° F.
Cut the squash in half (long-ways) and scrape out the seeds to "clean" the center.
Place the squash face-down on a greased baking pan. I like to use olive oil to grease the pan.
Put the squash in the oven for 45 minutes.
Halfway through baking, turn it over and sprinkle with salt and pepper.*
It's finished baking when a knife easily pierces through the skin.

*Note: you may eat the squash by scooping it out of the skin like the skin is a bowl for the squash, or you may scrape the squash meat out of the skin and serve it skin-free!*

Variation:
Before baking, you may try peeling the skin off of the butternut squash with a vegetable
  peeler.
Then cut the squash into cubes.
Toss the cubes into a bowl with 1 tbsp. olive oil, and sprinkle with salt and pepper.
Then pour the squash onto the baking sheet and bake in the oven (350 ° F.) for 30-45
  minutes, until tender.

*\*Feel free to sprinkle other seasonings on the squash for different flavors and gain the benefits of the healing energetic properties of the particular spice. There is more about this in the Wei recipe section. For example, you may try turmeric, cinnamon, rosemary, thyme, or Herbs de Provence. Have fun!*

CHINESE MEDICINE REFERENCES

**Butternut squash** — Another wonderful squash! Sweet and orange/yellow, it nourishes the earth element, stomach, and spleen/pancreas organs by moistening stomach yin and helping qi descend.

Baking foods puts heat into the food and concentrates the food - giving a kidney energy boost.

# Old-Fashioned Oatmeal

**Serves 2** | Cook time: 5 minutes or 15 minutes, depending on the type of oats

*My personal go-to for breakfast is watery oatmeal with a handful of mixed nuts and a few raisins on top and some almond milk. The watery oatmeal nourishes stomach yin. The nuts, including almond milk, provide protein and support the lungs. The raisins add sweetness and support kidney qi and nourish the blood.*

## INGREDIENTS

½ c. steel-cut oatmeal (quick-cooking, or regular)
2 c. water
⅓ c. nuts — your favorite kind (I like mixed nuts)
Optional — cinnamon, almond milk, ¼ c. raisins

## DIRECTIONS

Into a small saucepan, add the water and the oatmeal.
Bring to a boil, then reduce heat to simmer.
Stir the oats occasionally while on the stove top heat to help absorb the water.
When the oats are done, they won't be thirsty for more water.
Pour into 2 bowls.
Top with nuts.

*Note: If you are a purist and prefer the regular grains, it takes about 10-15 minutes to cook the oatmeal. If you are in a hurry, cook the quick-cooking oats, it will be about 5 minutes until ready to eat.*

---

CHINESE MEDICINE REFERENCES

**Oats** — They are so nourishing for the stomach. Eating them prepared in watery form nourishes stomach yin. Stomach yin is essential for the immune system and healthy digestion. Your stomach will notice the goodness you've given it very quickly, and it will relax!

**Cinnamon** — You may add a little cinnamon, especially if you feel a little chilly. It is a warming spice that is good for the heart and warms all the organs.

**Raisins** — These dried fruits contribute sweetness and nourish the blood and kidney qi.

**Nuts and Almond milk** — From the Wei and Yuan level nut milks provide protein with the grain — the perfect breakfast food combination!

# Congee, or Jook

**Serves 4-6  |  Cook time: 50-60 minutes**

*Congee is the staple breakfast food and snack food in China (it is called "jook" in Japan). It is a watery rice porridge used as a base for other foods that are placed on top. Making congee can be a meditative process if you are so inclined. Stirring the rice into the water can be a relaxing, focused activity. For that matter, all cooking can be meditative! (NOTE: See "Cooking and Eating as Meditation," pg. 26 for detailed guidance.)*

## INGREDIENTS

1 c. medium grain or long-grain white rice, washed, and in a large pot
10-12 c. water — boiling in a separate pot on the stove
1 tbsp. good oil (eg. grapeseed, or safflower, or organic peanut oil )
2 pinches of salt

*Note: Use good quality medium grain or long-grain white rice. Other varieties of rice don't work, they are too sticky. One cup of rice makes about 8-10 cups of congee, enough for 4-6 servings.*

## DIRECTIONS

Put 1 c. uncooked rice into a large pot.
Add 1 tbsp. oil and turn the heat on to high. Stir the rice in the oil, to coat each grain.
   Add a couple of pinches of salt.
After 2-3 minutes, add boiling water, enough to make the grains float (maybe a cup).
Stir constantly, the grains are absorbing the water.
When they have soaked up the liquid, gradually add more boiling water, and keep stirring.
After 3 or 4 more additions of water, stirring constantly for about 10 minutes, the grains
   will give up their starch to the water, called "first starch." The water will be milky-colored.
Now add a lot more water and bring down the heat to a gentle simmer for 30-40 minutes.
   You only need to stir occasionally at this stage, keeping the grains from settling and
   sticking to the bottom of the pot.
Add water as needed to keep the consistency at a milky water with very soft rice grains in it.

It's amazing how much water the rice will absorb! Congee is finished when it won't absorb any more water. If you leave it too long while it's simmering, congee will turn into a thick paste — meaning it still wants more water added. This is the water that gets absorbed in the digestive process — it is very helpful!

Serve congee with other things. If this is breakfast, please include protein, such as a sliced boiled egg or poached egg on top, or a little sliced fish. Chopped scallions or sliced ginger are typical additions, and cilantro, or bean sprouts. Using a high-quality soy sauce (or its kin, wheatless tamari sauce) makes a big difference in flavor. Keeping in mind what you need for your health, choose your additions with your knowledge of food energetics and wisdom.

---

CHINESE MEDICINE REFERENCES

**Congee Rice** — The watery consistency gets absorbed into the digestive tract, bringing nourishing yin fluids that our digestive tract craves for health. Rice is the most neutral grain, meaning it is the least allergic grain for most people. It nourishes the stomach qi. Typically, it is the first food for babies because it nourishes the stomach so gently. If you've had digestive issues, rice is often the best place to start to return health to your digestion.

**Grains** — Grains are the first food to nourish the stomach. This means that grains support digestion, especially grains cooked to be watery. Boiling foods brings water into the food. Adding water to foods is helpful for the stomach fluids (stomach yin), which enable digestion. One of the main causes of indigestion and digestive difficulties is that the stomach is too hot and dry. This means that the stomach gets stagnant, sluggish in its ability to process foods, which leads to discomfort and worse!

Having watery grains for breakfast is a nourishing way to start the day, and so delicious!

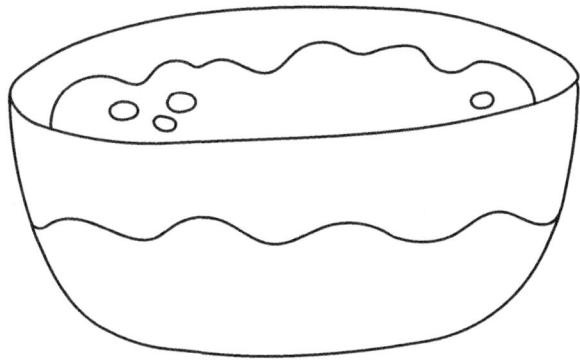

# wei recipes

Recipes in the Wei section focus on ingredients
that mostly come from high above the land or sky.

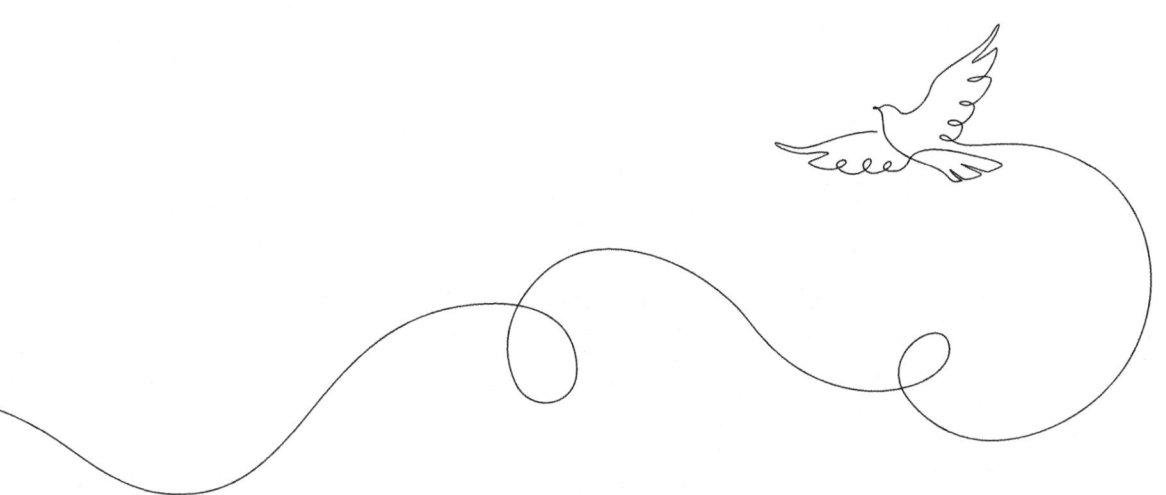

# Apple Pie

Serves 6-8   |   Prep time: 20 minutes prep   |   Cook time: 60 minutes baking

*This is a version of "pie" I prefer because it has less crust and more lightness. Wheat as a grain is warming and congesting, the gluten in it makes it "sticky" to digest. Instead of using wheat flour, this recipe uses almond flour and coconut flour, which are both nuts instead of grains.*

## INGREDIENTS

5-6 large tart apples (Granny Smiths are good)
¾ c. sugar
½ c. almond flour
½ c. coconut flour*
1 tsp. baking powder
1 beaten egg
1 tsp. vanilla
3-4 tbsp. melted coconut oil*

## DIRECTIONS

Preheat oven to 350° F.
Peel the apples and dice them.
Put the cut-up apples in a baking pan (a 9x9-inch baking pan works well).
Mix all dry ingredients.
Add the beaten egg and vanilla and mix into a lumpy dough.
Spread over the apples.
Pour oil over the top. Sprinkle generously with cinnamon.
Bake in the oven for about 1 hour, until golden brown.

*Variations:
You may substitute ½ c. gluten-free flour mix or wheat flour instead of the coconut flour, but I think the almond flour adds a very nice element to the flavor, so keep it in!
You may substitute melted butter instead of the coconut oil, use 6 tbsp. butter.

This recipe introduces the Wei level energy of food, because apples and nuts grow on trees, above earth, and influence the external layer of our body. Notice how some people who are allergic to nuts get skin irritations? The Wei level has to do with the surface of the body, the skin. Most foods people are allergic to come from either Yuan or Wei levels. Wei level allergies tend to show up on the skin (the Wei level) while most Yuan level allergies show up deeper in the body (such as internal swelling), at the Yuan level.

**Apples** — Apples, and most fruit, are cooling energetically, and therefore harder on the stomach to digest. By baking the apples (adding heat) and adding cinnamon, the overall quality of the recipe is balanced, not too cool, and easy to digest.

**Cinnamon** — This is a Wei-level aromatic spice. Most spices are Wei level, especially those that are aromatic.

**Vanilla** — This is also a Wei-level aromatic, vanilla relaxes the heart.

# Embodied Eating Experience

*Notice the difference in how the fruit feels in your mouth raw, or baked, or baked with butter and honey or sugar? It tends to feel refreshing raw or baked, but when butter and honey or sugar are added, something different takes place. Do you feel the added heat and stickiness of the butter and honey or sugar? The sweetness is intensified, and so is the coagulation ability of the fruit and sauce now. You may even experience a stuffy nose or nasal congestion after eating fruit prepared with butter and honey or sugar!*

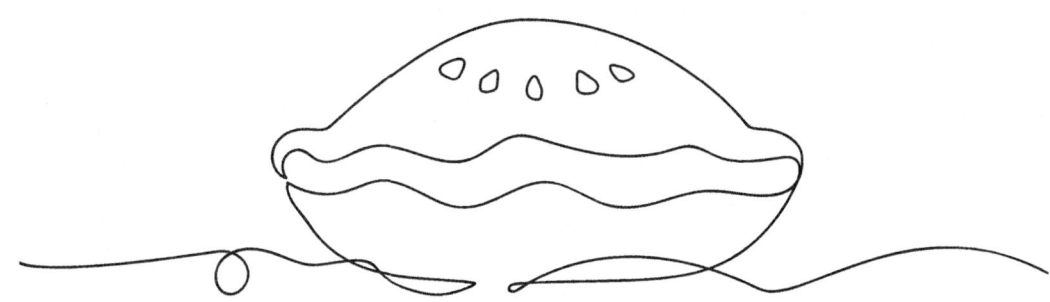

# Baked Fruit Desserts

Serves as many people as you have fruit for!
Prep time: 5-10 minutes
Cook time: 40-50 minutes, preheating the oven may be the most time-consuming part!

o————————————————————————————————————o

*Simple, sweet fruit makes the best desserts, in my humble opinion. It's easy to transform them from their off-the-tree goodness into dinner-guest specialness. Here are a few variations of baked fruit. Slow roasting them saves tart under-ripe fruit, turning them into delicious desserts.*

## INGREDIENTS

4 apples or 4 pears or 8 plums or 4 peaches (Or a combination of these! Plan for one half or one whole piece of fruit per person or 1-2 plums per person.)
Brown sugar or honey to taste

## DIRECTIONS

Preheat oven to 400° F.

Wash 4 apples, and remove the core. Fill the hole from the core with brown sugar or honey. Set in a baking pan and roast in the oven for 30-40 minutes, until soft and tender.

or

Wash 4 pears, cut them in half, and remove the cores. Fill the hole from the core with brown sugar or honey. Set them in a baking pan in a single layer, cut side up. Bake for 30-40 minutes, until tender and juicy.

or

Wash 8 plums, slice in half, and remove the pits. Fill the hole from the pits with brown sugar or honey. Set them in a baking pan in a single layer, cut side up. Bake for 30-45 minutes, until tender and juicy.

or

Wash 4 peaches, slice in half, and remove pits. Fill the hole from the pits with brown sugar or honey. Set them in a baking pan in a single layer, sliced side up. Bake for 30-40 minutes, until tender and juicy.

*Optional for special occasions:*
Prepare the fruit of choice as above. Before setting the fruit in a baking dish, melt 4 tbsp. butter in the pan (in the oven), then sprinkle 1 c. brown sugar over the butter. Then place the fruit cut side down on the pan. Bake for 30-40 minutes. Turn fruit over, baste with the pan sauce, and bake 10 minutes more, until glossy. Allow to cool slightly before serving. Sprinkling with sliced almonds is an elegant touch.

**Fruit** — Fruit is the reproductive goal of the tree or bush. (The same is true for nuts and seeds.) The seeds or pit embedded deep inside contain the genetic code for the plant's potential for full growth. Fruit grows on the tree branch, living on the exterior regions, the Wei qi level. Fruits tend to invigorate the qi and the blood. Fruits are also cold in nature, so we need to be careful about eating them since the stomach does not digest well when we eat "cold" foods. If you feel like you are catching a cold, do not eat fruit! Baking fruit intensifies the sweetness and brings out the qualities the fruit offers. For example, pears are cooling and moistening to the body, even when their ambient temperature is warm from the oven. All tree fruit nourishes the upper and outer level of the body energetic, the Wei level. This means that tree fruit, growing out of the flowers of the tree and then falling to the ground when ripe, brings energy from above to below. Physically, this means moving the energy of the lungs, guiding it down through the body, through the intestines.

**Honey** — Honey comes from pollen, which comes from flowers, and is gathered by bees. There is a lot going into this nectar that is the result of the plant's reproductive expression (flower) and the bees' reproductive activity (pollen turning to honey in the hive for the queen). Honey is a potent food! It is very healing for allergies. If local honey is eaten by local allergy sufferers, a small amount of honey daily can help the body build immunity to the local pollens. Of course, its sweetness cannot be matched by anything else, and its flavor varies according to the flowers the bees visited to collect pollen.

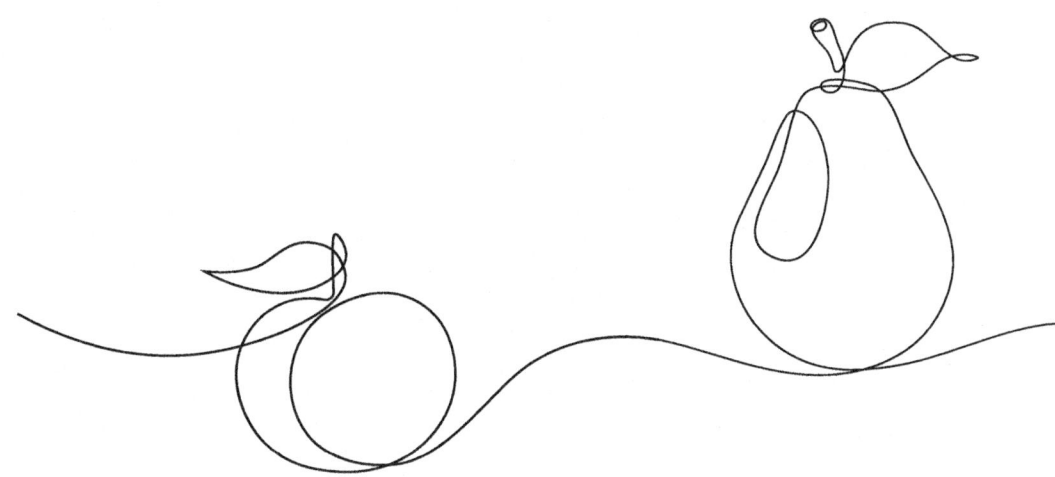

# Mimi's Best Granola

**Makes 12-15 servings  |  Prep time: 15 minutes**

*My dear friend, Mimi, created this recipe for her family. When her kids came home from college, they devoured it! Now it is a requested gift whenever Mimi visits her kids. My family loves it, too. Thanks, Mimi!*

## INGREDIENTS

1 c. each: walnuts, pecans, macadamia nuts, cashews, and slivered almonds
⅓ c. each: sunflower seeds and pumpkin seeds
⅓ c. combined hemp, chia, and flax seeds
3 tsp. each: cinnamon and vanilla
⅓ c. maple syrup
3 c. oats

## DIRECTIONS

Combine all ingredients in a large bowl, adding the syrup and vanilla last, mix well.
The best way to get the benefit of the oats is to soak the granola overnight. You may put 1 c. of the granola in a bowl, pour water to cover it and set it in the refrigerator overnight. In the morning, take it out of the fridge, and allow it to come to room temperature before eating. I like to pour almond milk over the top for breakfast. You may roast the nuts and oats separately in a pan on the stove top to increase the yang (warming and moving) energy in the food.

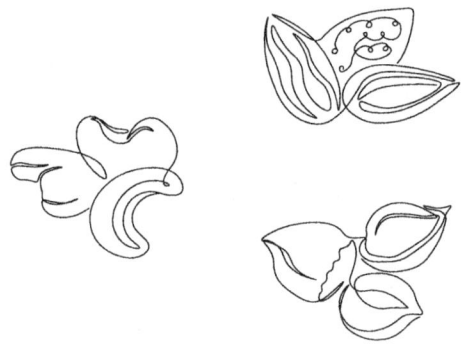

**Oats** — Oats are a non-glutinous grain that nourishes the stomach organ. Oats heal inflammation and cool heat in the digestive tract. They also help reduce cholesterol. I've talked about the wonders of whole grains in the section about porridge. This is another way to enjoy the benefits of oats: as granola!

**Nuts and seeds** — This recipe includes a variety of nuts. Nuts and seeds are the reproductive products of their plant or tree. As such, they nourish the deep Yuan level, the essence, constitutional level of the body, supporting kidney energy. They also grow on trees, above the earth, supporting the Wei level, the lungs, immune system, and skin. Interestingly, most allergies happen from foods at the Wei and/or Yuan levels.

**Almonds and pine nuts** — bitter and descend the energy, good for helping resolve constipation, belonging to the metal element, supporting the lungs and large intestines.

**Walnuts** — good for the brain. They even look like brains when shelled!

**Pecans** — high in fat, and support the liver (as do Brazil nuts and Walnuts).

**Cashews** — good for the kidney energy, water element, (along with peanuts, chestnuts and walnuts).

**Macadamia nuts and Hazelnuts** — good for the earth element, the stomach, pancreas/spleen.

**Pistachios** — aka "the happiness nuts" because they ascend qi to the chest, relaxing the heart.

**Pumpkin seeds** — help with many digestive issues and are good for the stomach, spleen/pancreas.

**Sunflower seeds** — help make phlegm move. Sunflowers follow the sun; they store yang qi. Sunflower and safflower oil are not good to use if you have inflammation. It's better to use olive oil, or avocado oil instead.

**Poppy seeds** — some of the tiniest seeds we eat, have an affinity to the heart. They lift depression, reaching the kidney qi and bringing it up to relax and open the heart.

**Chia seeds** — these little seeds reach the liver, and heart and kidney qi. They clear heat in the blood that can manifest as nervous anxiety, and irritability.

**Vanilla** — This spice is a Wei-level food. When you get a whiff of vanilla scent, you simply sigh "ahh"— the sound of the heart relaxing. Vanilla relaxes the heart, opening the heart for more self-expression.

**Cinnamon** — This spice warms the body, it enters every organ channel, supporting the immune system.

**Maple syrup** — This sweet, sticky elixir contains the signature of the sap, the lifeblood, of the tree. Sap rises up from the roots to the leaves, communicating the uplifting message of growth to the tree, and then it moves back down the trunk to the roots, up and down in a rhythm of integration of the tree's essence and purpose — to grow toward heaven.

What a wonderful way to start the day! With a relaxed and open heart, warm and nourished kidney essence, and oats to fortify and circulate the energy of digestion, and inspiration!

# Almond Milk

**Serves 3-4 (1 cup/each)**  |  **Prep time: 10 minutes after soaking nuts for 8-10 hours overnight**

*Nut milks are so easy to make. Try it and you might never buy nut milk again! Buy nuts that are kept in the refrigerated section of the store; and never, ever use any that smell stale or rancid!*

## INGREDIENTS

1 c. almonds (or cashews, sunflower seeds, etc.)
3-4 c. water
You'll also need:
cheesecloth
blender

## DIRECTIONS

Bathe the raw nuts or seeds in enough cool water to cover them.
Soak overnight — you may leave them out on your kitchen counter.
In the morning, discard the soaking water, rinse and drain them.
Put the softened nuts or seeds in your blender.
Slowly add water and blend until smooth.
Pour the mixture into a cheesecloth over a clean basin and drain. Now you have almond milk!

*Note: If the milk is too thick, add more water. It will keep in the refrigerator for a few days. And, you may save the nut solids to use in baking, if you like.*

CHINESE MEDICINE REFERENCES

**Nut and Seed Milk** — This tasty milk nourishes kidney yin in a very strong way. It clears heat, calms stress, and opens the heart. You may select the nut or seeds based on the specific properties that each one holds and what you need. Note: These properties are discussed in Mimi's Best Granola, pg. 97.

# Simple Citrus Dressing

**Makes 1 cup of dressing  |  Prep time: 10 minutes**

*This is an elegant, light dressing for a summer salad. Although TCM does not favor eating cold, raw food, an occasional raw salad is lovely, especially in the hot summertime. Chewing crunchy foods stimulates the digestive juices, aiding the stomach.*

## INGREDIENTS

1 lemon
1 orange
1 lime
¼ c. olive oil
salt
pepper

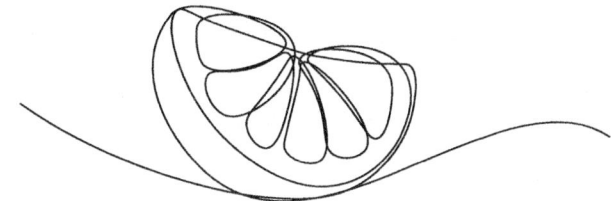

## DIRECTIONS

Cut the fruit in half.
In a small bowl, combine equal parts of fresh, squeezed fruit juices and olive oil —
  ¼ c. lemon juice, ¼ c. orange juice, and ¼ c. lime juice with ¼ c. olive oil.
Add about 1 tsp. salt and add pepper to taste, maybe just ¼ tsp. pepper.
Stir all ingredients together with a fork, whisking vigorously until blended.
Carefully add more salt if needed — not enough salt and the dressing will be bitter. Too
  much salt and it will be too salty tasting. Add just the right amount, and the sweetness
  of the juices comes out, it's delicious!

CHINESE MEDICINE REFERENCES

**Dressing** — The olive oil is slightly bitter. The lemon and lime juice is sour, while the orange is sweet. The salt brings it all together. The pepper adds a little heat. A perfectly balanced combination of the Five Elements of flavors!

# Gingerbread Cake

Serves 12 | Prep time : 20 minutes | Cook time: 45-50 minutes

*This is a wonderful, dairy-free cake! You may bake it gluten free, too. When my kids were on a high school ski team, the coach's parents would show up in their trailer and the kids would pile in there to warm up and have hot chocolate and treats. Perhaps it was their favorite part of being on the ski team! A couple of the kids had dairy and gluten allergies, so I would bring this cake and it was always eaten up. It is our family's favorite cake in the winter time.*

## INGREDIENTS

1 c. sugar
¾ c. canola oil
1 c. dark molasses
2 tsp. baking soda
2 ¾ c. flour - or Bob's Red Mill 1 to 1 Baking flour
½ tsp. sea salt
1 tsp. ground ginger
½ tsp. ground cinnamon
½ tsp. ground cloves
2 large eggs, beaten

## DIRECTIONS

Preheat oven to 350 degrees F.

Oil a 9x12 inch baking pan, line the bottom of the pan with parchment paper, oil the parchment.

Combine the sugar, oil, and molasses in a large mixing bowl. Dissolve the baking soda in 1 c. boiling water (it will fizz!). Sift together the flour, spices, and salt. Stir the dry mixture into the wet one. Gently beat the eggs into the mix, use a whisk or electric beater on low. Mix until just combined, no lumps of flour.

Pour the batter into the pan. Bake for about 45 minutes, until a toothpick inserted into the center of the cake comes out clean.

Cool before cutting. A little fresh whipped cream on top makes it extra special. (But I like it plain).

**Molasses** — is made from boiling and then concentrating sugar cane. It's mild sweetness supports Stomach and Spleen/Pancreas, and it nourishes the blood.

**Ginger** — is a root and aids digestion, especially nausea and bloating.

**Cinnamon** — is warming and helps prevent stagnation (especially good for digesting sweet desserts).

**Cloves** — are hot.

**Spices** — are very warming, and aromatic. All of these spices support the Stomach and Spleen/Pancreas, Liver/Gallbladder, and Small Intestines. They are so potent for treating cold in the digestive tract that they are used in our TCM pharmacy! The heat in these spices also supports Kidney yang which, among many things, helps to maintain body warmth.

Baking as a cooking technique puts heat into the food. All of these factors make this cake especially tempting (and helpful) in cold weather!

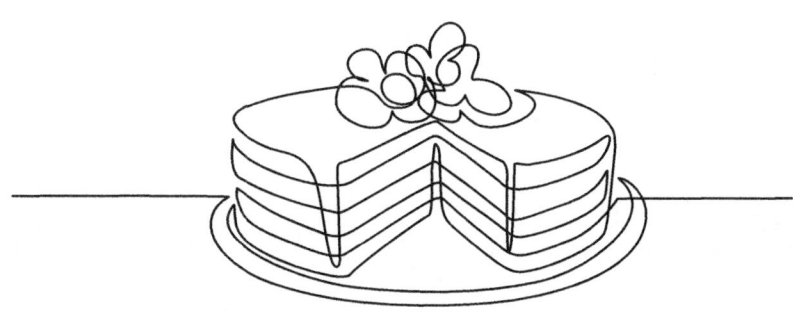

# Simple Trail Mix

**Serves 8** | **Prep time 10 minutes**

## INGREDIENTS

1 c. almonds
1 c. pecans
1 c. cashews
½ c. dried apricots - diced small
½ c. dried plums (prunes) - diced small
¼ c. coconut flakes

## DIRECTIONS

In a large bowl, mix all ingredients together and enjoy! You may also divide the mixture into ½ cup servings and store ready to go into lunchboxes. Store in an airtight container up to 3-4 weeks.

If you'd like to add more warmth (to support kidney energy) to the mix, put the nuts in a dry pan on the stove and heat them up, moving them around in the pan so they don't burn. When you smell the nutty delicious fragrance -they are done. Allow them to cool before adding the other ingredients.

---

CHINESE MEDICINE REFERENCES

**Prunes and apricots** — are major movers of qi for the intestines- they treat constipation and food stagnation. If you tend to diarrhea this mix would be too much, don't eat it! Plums and apricots, like almost all fruits, are cooling. However, drying them adds warmth, aiding digestion.

**Almonds, cashews, pecans** — are all descending, drawing on lung qi (Wei level) to help direct qi downwards.

**Coconut** — is cooling and hydrating

---

# appendices

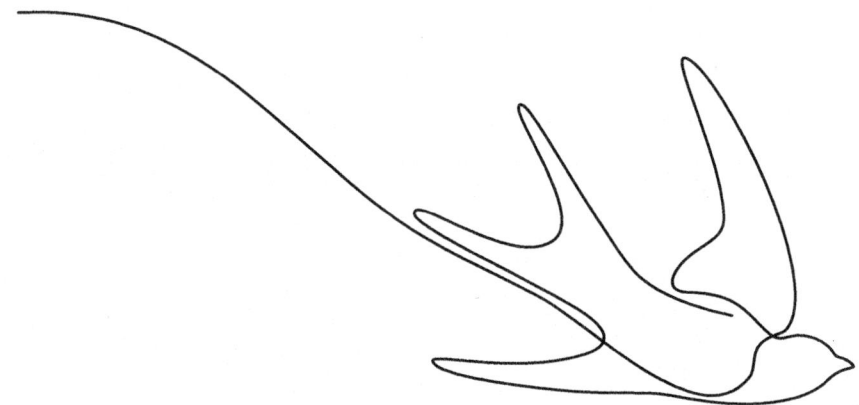

## MEAL SUGGESTIONS & PAIRINGS

Here are a few ways to think about putting together meals with consideration of Yin/Yang; the 3 levels of Yuan, Ying, and Wei; and the Five Elements.

### Breakfast:

Basic Meal: Grain + Protein
- Oatmeal (pg. 87) + nuts + Almond Milk (pg. 98)
- Congee (pg. 88) + sardines
- Congee (pg. 88) + hard or soft boiled egg or scrambled eggs with chives, scallions or thyme
- Oatmeal (pg. 87) + pork breakfast sausage, ham, bacon or chicken breakfast sausage
- Mimi's Best Granola (pg. 96) + Almond Milk (pg. 98)

### Lunch and Dinner:

Basic Meal: Grain (or root vegetable) + Green/Yellow Vegetables + Protein

*Protein: Vegetarian vs. Carnivore?*

This is a BIG topic, but here are a few brief thoughts:
- Without a doubt, the world would benefit from a reduction in meat consumption — even reducing 1/3 the amount of meat eaten would make a difference for our planet environmentally.
- Another part of the issue with eating meat is the way that animals are raised and treated. This can lead to vegetarianism for ethical or sympathetic reasons — or for health reasons — all very good reasons.
- Animal protein is healthy protein, containing fat, which is necessary for the brain and hormones to function. New research shows that cardiovascular health has more to do with stress than eating red meat! When we eat animal meat, we are taking in the energy of that particular animal. In our modern society, we can still benefit from the Yang energy of animals.
- We need to balance the warming and cooling qualities of food for health. Animal meat is warming or hot, so not eating too much is important, and eating vegetables with it is important. Eating only plants tends to be too cooling, so including warming spices and consuming high-quality fats (such as fat from nuts and high-quality butter and plant oils) is important for vegetarian and vegan diets.

Here are some suggestions for balanced meals from this book:

*Note: Pairings listed with a "V" are vegetarian and/or vegan*
- Broiled Salmon (pg. 38) + Moroccan Carrots (pg. 76) + Roasted Broccoli (pg. 68)
- Greek Lemon Artichoke Chicken (pg. 54) + rice + Braised Chard (pg. 64) + Baked Butternut Squash (pg. 86)
- Smoked Trout (or Salmon ) w/Warm Potato Salad (pg. 40) + Roasted Chard or Kale (pg. 72) + Sautéed Zucchini (pg. 84)
- Chicken Soup (pg. 46), add 1 c. of washed rice
- Manx Lamb Stew (pg. 60)
- Cottage Pie (pg. 52) + Sautéed Mushrooms (pg. 44)
- Spatchcocked Chicken (pg. 56) + Eiko's Sesame Spinach (pg. 66) + Roasted Delicata Squash & Sage (pg. 82)
- Sausage & Bean Soup (pg. 48) + hearty whole-grain bread
- Broiled Salmon (pg. 38) + Roasted Root Vegetables (pg. 77) + Stewed Okra (pg. 74)
- Spinach Rice with Shrimp (pg. 42), Barbecued Yellow Squash (pg. 85)
- V – Stuffed Spaghetti Squash (pg. 80) + quinoa, lentils
- V – Bean & Vegetable Chili (pg. 62) + quinoa or rice
- V – Split-Pea Soup (pg. 50) + hearty whole-grain bread
- V – Smoky Lentil Stew (pg. 58) + rice

To make dinner special, serve **dessert!** Try:
- V – Baked Fruit Desserts (pg. 94)
- V – Apple Pie (pg. 92)
- V – Gingerbread Cake (pg. 100)

## FOOD & ORGAN AFFINITIES

There are 8 categories of food. Broadly, foods from the plant and animal kingdoms have affiliations with the Five Element organ systems within the three dimensions of Yuan, Ying, and Wei. These are associations, and some foods have an affinity to more than one organ and element:

### Grain and Vegetables

Plants, or vegetables in general, are associated with the wood element, but may be further broken down:

- Grains — Grains nourish the earth element, and thus, the stomach, pancreas, and spleen.
- Green vegetables — mainly support the liver/gallbladder and wood element. Most descend the qi, but the stalks (asparagus, celery, etc.) ascend qi.
- Sprouts — grow upward and are diuretics.
- Broad Leafy — opens and spreads the qi (spinach, chard, kale, collards).
- Legumes — beans, cooling for stomach yin, support kidneys and liver/gallbladder (lentils, black beans, kidney beans, lima, cannelli, pinto, etc.).
- Bitter Greens — very cooling, strongly descending (endive, radicchio, dandelion greens, turnip greens, broccoli rabe, etc.).
- Yellow vegetables — squashes - easy to digest, support stomach, spleen/pancreas/ small intestine (zucchini, butternut, acorn, delicata, yellow summer squash, spaghetti ).
- Root vegetables — move qi downward (carrots, parsnips, rutabaga, beets, turnips, etc.).
- Tubers — consolidate qi to the center, nourishing stomach, spleen/pancreas, liver/ gallbladder (sweet potato, yam, white potato, cassava root).
- Fermented foods — aid digestion by supplying "starters" (digestive microbes) for the process, downward moving, support stomach, spleen/pancreas (sauerkraut, kombucha, miso, kimchee, yogurt, tofu).
- A word about tofu — made from fermented soy (as is miso), it is very cooling, and so some people have difficulty digesting it. It is often cooked with warming spices and sauces to balance this issue. The other problem is that soy is used a lot in processed foods and has been linked to hormone disruption.  Please avoid soy (and tofu) that is used in processed foods.
- Mushrooms, seaweeds, and seeds — These plants nourish the water element, which includes the kidneys and urinary bladder.

### Fruits

Fruits, in general, are cooling and nourish the lungs and metal element at the Wei level.

- Pit fruits, such as plums, apricots, cherries also tend to be useful as meat tenderizers when cooked with meats.
- Fruits that grow on bushes or the ground, such as blueberries, blackberries, strawberries, have an affinity for the wood element, liver/gallbladder organs, and tend to nourish the blood.

- Compact fruits - apples, pears- have edible skins, affiliated with the metal element.
- Tropical fruits have inedible skins - pineapple, coconut, banana - and have earth element affinity.
- Citrus fruits are diuretics, and connected to the water element.
- Melons grow on vines close to the ground, an affinity to stomach and spleen/pancreas.

## Nuts and Seeds

Seeds have an affinity to the kidneys and water element at the Yuan level. Nuts, especially that come from trees, are from the Wei level. Foods can have affinity for more than one category. For a detailed look at nut and seed organ affiliations see page 97.

## Flowers

The heart represents the fire organ — it goes with flowers, vanilla, and saffron. The heart is thought of as being the sovereign of the body (and the human being). As sovereign, it needs very little, and very few foods nourish the fire element. Its purpose is to provide — to give us life, wisdom, and joy.

## Meat

Meats that come from the land are very warming. Meats from the sea (fish) tend to be relatively cooling, but that can change with cooking methods. They can be further broken down into organ affiliations:
- Beef, veal, and buffalo — These meats have an affinity with the wood element and the liver.
- Chicken and poultry — These have an affinity with the earth element and the stomach, pancreas, and spleen.
- Freshwater fish, turkey, and lamb — These meats have an affinity with the metal element and the lungs.
- Pork, shellfish, ocean fish, duck, and bones of animals (as in bone broth) — These all have an affinity with the water element and the kidneys.
- Turkey — Turkey has an affinity with the fire element and heart, as it calms the heart.

## Dairy

Eggs and milk, the reproductive materials of the animal, are associated primarily with the kidneys, and the Yuan level. But they are also affiliated with the Wei level, since both eggs and milk are expressed from the animal and come out to the surface, these are Wei level attributes. It is interesting that most food allergies come from either the Yuan level or the Wei level. There are few allergens that come from the Ying level. We depend on the Ying level to provide the staple foods — grains, greens, and proteins (both meat and beans).

## Warming & Cooling Aspects

Foods may also be classified as being more warming or cooling energetically:

• Foods from the Yuan level, associated with the kidneys, tend to be more cooling.
• Foods from the Ying level, associated with liver, stomach, pancreas, and spleen, are more warming.
• Foods associated with the Wei level tend to be both warming (bringing the energy out to the surface) and also cooling (bringing relief to the surface if the body is too hot).
• Eggs and milk tend to be warming, and are classified at the Yuan level, as well as the Wei level.
• Cooking methods contribute qi to foods.
• Steaming and boiling exposes food to water, adding yin.
• Grilling and roasting foods adds heat from below, while broiling adds heat from above, spreading heat out.
• Baking food concentrates the heat. Frying food subjects the food to fat.


[APPENDIX C]

# FLAVORS & CRAVINGS

Each of the five flavors is associated with an element system in the body. This means that each organ and its realm of influence responds to particular flavors, and may require particular flavors, for nourishment. So when an element is in need, one way it cries out for help is by craving a particular flavor. Risking oversimplification, here is a quick connection between flavors and organs.

## Salty

The salty flavor is associated with the water element and the kidney organ system. The kidney qi governs the endocrine system, bones and bone marrow, and the water system (urinary system) in the body. If kidney qi gets stressed somehow, one way it sends out a distress signal is to crave the salty flavor. The adrenal glands are a part of the kidney system (they sit on top of each kidney) and a classic sign of adrenal fatigue is craving salt. Salt craving may be a sign that you need more rest.

## Sweet

If the earth element, which is the stomach and digestive system, is distressed it craves the sweet flavor. Among its many responsibilities for digestion, the stomach funds mental concentration. A common result of overthinking, or worry, is to crave sweets. This may be a sign that there is a need to relax the mind. When the stomach and digestive system are functioning very well, then the sweet flavor, in balance with all the other flavors, nourishes the stomach. When they are not functioning well, sweet is a problem. Think about diabetes and what sweets do to the pancreas/digestive system.

## Bitter

The heart and cardiovascular system are connected with the fire element and the bitter flavor. We associate dark chocolate's slightly bitter flavor with the heart; it's more than a Valentine's Day affiliation! Coffee has a bitter tone, and it affects the heart, too. Think about drinking too much coffee and your heart pumping faster as a result! If we crave bitter flavor, it may be a sign the heart and cardiovascular system need attention. If this system is functioning very well, then a balanced amount of the bitter flavor nourishes the system.

## Sour

The wood element is associated with the liver, the gallbladder, and the detoxification system. The liver produces bile, a very sour flavor. Craving sour things, such as sucking on a lemon, or eating dill pickles or green olives, means the liver system is being addressed. The liver also governs the smooth flow of emotional energy. When we feel frustrated or angry, it may stimulate wanting something sour. A little sour also activates the liver to aid good digestion.

## Spicy, Pungent

The metal element is affiliated with the lungs and respiratory system and the spicy, pungent flavor. If people crave very spicy, robust flavor, it may be that they need to clear their chest, or breathe more easily — physically and/or emotionally! A balanced amount of this flavor activates the lung and respiratory system, giving nourishment to its function. Too much may create many various problems; an obvious one is coughing when eating very spicy foods!

## Bland

There is a sixth flavor, called "bland." Bland does not mean "no flavor!" It is the gentle, more subtle flavor, and it can be very helpful to aid digestion. The small intestine has a special affinity for bland flavor foods. Think of Cantonese cooking like Moo Goo Gai Pan; the flavors are subtle and delicious. A lot of these dishes are based on steamed vegetables (zucchini, okra, etc.) and tofu. Another example would be tapioca pudding. This flavor soothes the small intestine and the entire digestive system. It is important as a diet remedy for healing various gut problems because it is clearing. When a person needs digestive cures, a clear, bland diet is often a first step.

## Got a flavor craving?

It is good to seek medical attention from a Traditional Chinese Medicine doctor for an accurate diagnosis if strong craving for any flavor persists. There can be a complex root reason as to why certain cravings exist, and a TCM doctor will know how best to go about treatment.

## NOURISHING THE IMMUNE SYSTEM

Nourishing the immune system, or "Defensive Qi", is an important part of good health. Here are basic tips on how to do this. The big components of Defensive Qi are:
- **Kidney Yang:** the warming, activating energy that protects us
- **Stomach Yin:** the deep hydration that moistens the gut and keeps it healthy
- **Lung Qi:** the respiratory system energy is about our interaction with the external world. Obviously, it includes the breath, but it also includes the skin, our outermost layer that protects us from harmful influences.

### DEFENSIVE QI DOS AND DON'TS

### Kidney Yang

**Don'ts/depleters:** Think of Kidney energy as the bank account for the body. We want to have a big savings account and keep depositing into it — not making withdrawals — in order to build up our immune system. These things drain the kidney energy "savings," so avoid:
- Cold, raw foods, and "sticky" foods: sugar, dairy, and gluten.
- Artificial stimulants — coffee, chocolate, hot spices, garlic, onion, sugar, alcohol, and "recreational" drugs.
- Electronic equipment (including phones) in the bedroom.

**Dos:** These things nourish, or make contributions to, Kidney Yang, so:
- Sleep! Go to bed before 10:00 p.m.
- Rest! Nap if you are tired.
- Eat regular meals to get energy from the food you eat — do not fast which draws on the kidney energy reserves.
- Treasure and cultivate calm — meditate and practice qigong!

**Stomach Yin**

**Don'ts/depleters:** Think of the Stomach as a big cooking pot, simmering on the stove. We want the pot to always have moisture in it, never drying out as it is simmering. These things dry out the stomach energy, so **avoid**:
- Dehydrating foods — coffee, chocolate, hot spices, garlic, onion, sugar, alcohol, and carbonated drinks.
- Inflammatory foods — GMOs, pesticides, known allergens, sugar, dairy, yeast, soy, alcohol, and vinegars.

**Dos:** These things nourish Stomach Yin, keeping the moisture inside, so:
- Eat wet foods — watery porridge for breakfast, soups, stews, broths, and casseroles.
- Eat a little saturated fat — butter, eggs, fish, and animal fat.
- Rest when digesting.
- Sleep! Go to bed before 10:00 p.m.

**Lung qi**

**Don'ts/Depleters:** Think of Lung Qi as how we physically meet the external world: with our skin and our breath, so **avoid**:
- Congesting foods — sugar, gluten, and dairy are the most sticky and therefore, most difficult to digest and can congest the lungs/sinus.
- Holding your breath or shallow breathing.
- Getting cold — especially the back of your neck.

**Dos:** To meet the external world, be full of your own Qi! Be happy!
- Breathe! Take slow, deep, relaxed breaths throughout the day, practice until this is the way you naturally breathe.
- Wash your hands regularly, wash your body daily.
- Keep your body temperature warm and well regulated.
- Have a good, deep belly laugh every day, even for no reason.

## ENERGETICS OF DIGESTION: YOUR HEALTH IS TIED TO YOUR STOMACH

*Note: Physically, the pancreas and spleen are so close together, they seem connected. Maybe this is how the Chinese Medicine translation of spleen ("pi") was assigned to the function of the pancreas. This has created some confusion over the years. So when I use the phrase "spleen" or "spleen qi," I am referring to the energetic functions of both the spleen and the pancreas organs.*

While many of us are very familiar with the digestive process as it's described in Western medicine, Chinese Medicine links digestion with energy (qi). This connects the health of your whole body with what happens in your stomach. These are two very different approaches!

Western medicine says a healthy digestive process looks like this:
- **Mouth:** The smell of food stimulates the salivary glands in your mouth to produce saliva, and you experience your mouth watering. When you chew food very well, your saliva breaks down the food while it's in your mouth.
- **Esophagus:** Next, you swallow the food down your esophagus. Your esophagus empties the food into your stomach.
- **Stomach:** Stomach chemicals (hydrochloric acid is the main one) break down the food even more. When the food in the stomach is small enough, it moves into the small intestine to be further broken down and sorted out.
- **Intestines:** The first third of the small intestine digests proteins, the second third digests grains, and the last third digests fruits and vegetables (roughage). There are hormones that are secreted from the stomach and small intestine that invite the pancreas, spleen, liver, and gallbladder to participate in digestion. When the small intestine is finished digesting food, it passes on the indigestible substances (fiber and water) to the large intestine to be eliminated (pooped out).

While the Western medicine description of healthy digestion is somewhat linear, the Chinese Medicine description is much more complex. Every organ is in communication with other organs. Digestion involves every organ system, including the emotions. What we eat, how we eat, when we eat, and how strong the stomach and spleen qi are all influence the subsequent flow of digestion. And after the stomach and spleen qi have facilitated digestion, the entire body receives nourishing Qi and Blood as a result. The health of the organs directly involves emotional health. To Chinese Medicine, emotions come from the organs and the brain receives the emotional information and names it. But we first feel in our "guts!"

***Chinese Medicine says a healthy digestive system functions like this:***
Digestion begins when the mouth takes in food, and the jaw moves with chewing, and we swallow fluids and food. In the stomach they begin to be broken down. The stomach is the source of body fluids.

Then, the stomach sends the semi-digested food and fluids to the spleen. The spleen qi transforms fluids and food into "food qi." That's right, the food you put in your body is transformed into food energy! Food qi gets further refined through the digestive process. Food qi transforms into nutritive qi. Nutritive qi is extracted from food and water and nourishes the interior of the body, all of the organs, tissues, and blood. Food qi also transforms into defensive qi. Defensive qi protects the skin and muscles, the body's exterior, which is the first layer of defense in the immune system.

## Functions of the Stomach and Spleen/Pancreas
The following is a list of functions of the Stomach and Spleen that are involved in transforming food into Food qi:
  - Stomach receives food and begins digestion
  - Stomach qi moves the flow of digestion downward
  - Spleen qi transforms food into Food qi
  - Spleen qi ascends Food qi to the chest, where it is refined and nourishes the lungs and the heart, then, it is transformed into blood.
  - Spleen qi transports Food qi to nourish all the body's tissues, especially muscles
  - Spleen qi transforms Food qi into Nutritive qi and Defensive qi
  - Spleen qi holds the blood in the blood vessels
  - Spleen qi lifts the organs, preventing prolapse
  - Spleen Yang qi warms the body
  - Spleen qi influences our ability to study, concentrate, and memorize

This is why the quality of food is paramount to Chinese Medicine!

## The Stomach, Spleen and the Digestive System
Problems with digestion begin when the stomach and spleen are overburdened by the wrong kinds of food, or inadequately chewed food, or too much food at one time, or food eaten too soon after the last ingestion. The other influence on digestion is emotional — when we feel very anxious or worried about what life will bring, the stomach and spleen qi contracts and we lose our appetite, or cannot digest what we have already eaten, or cannot feel satisfied. We will experience signs of stomach and spleen qi stagnation — digestive discomfort. The stomach takes in food, as well as life experiences and our emotional response to life experiences! When all is well, and stomach qi and spleen qi are flowing freely, we feel comfortable in our physical digestive process and we move through our life experiences with confidence and thoughtfulness toward others; we feel hungry for life (and food) and ready for more!

Eventually the stomach breaks down food into small enough particles to pass on to the small intestine. The first part of the small intestine is hot with stomach acid (yang), but most of the small intestine needs a cool, alkaline environment in order to function well. If the environment is too warm or damp (because of the difficult food conditions mentioned above), then extra energy is required from the stomach and spleen to assist — they send out cooling insulin and other digestive chemicals to the small intestine. If the need to step up the help persists, over time the stomach and spleen tire, creating bigger problems.

The small intestine sorts out foods for digestion — proteins, grains, and roughage (vegetables and fruits). The small intestine also sorts out information in life. Can we sort through all of the information we receive in order to find what is worthy of taking in, and what to bypass? Can we distinguish between experiences that are high-quality for our soul's nourishment and those that bring us down? Our ability to separate out the "pure" from the "impure" in order to deeply nourish our life is the deeper energy of the small intestine. If we find we are confused about truth and lies, or feel cynical, pessimistic, or negative, it is likely that the small intestine lacks enough qi in order to do a good job in sorting out our life experience.

The small intestine refines Nutritive qi. And it passes any remaining indigestible matter to the large intestine. The large intestine has the honor of receiving material from the small intestine and having the final decision on extracting any remaining value/nutrition from what it is given — and eliminating what is truly waste. When large intestine qi is abundant, bowel movements are easy and complete. If we find we struggle with holding on to stinky experiences and we can't let go of our feelings, it may be that the large intestine energy is stuck or weak. When we are able to let go of what no longer serves us and open to what is new, the large intestine energy is healthy.

Basically, when the digestive system is healthy, the energy of all the corresponding organ systems is functioning very well. When the digestive system is not healthy, then many different organs' energies may become imbalanced and sick. Let's explore how the organs respond to Nutritive qi, and how our emotions are an integral part of the organ systems. Our emotions and the health of their corresponding organ influence each other. We think of the organs as being members of one family. We met the first family members — the digestive system. Now let's meet the other four.

**The Lungs and Respiratory System**
Food qi ascends to the chest and nourishes the lungs and respiratory system, including the sinuses and skin. If the Food qi is clean, then the sinuses and skin are clear. If the Food qi is "damp," then we have sinus congestion. This directly influences the immune system, the defensive qi. In the emotional dimension, when the energy of the lungs is congested we experience sadness and grief. Also, these feelings constrict the energy of the lungs. When the lungs and respiratory system energy are free, we experience compassion easily. The lungs breathe, and the energy of their breath is integrated into food qi and then passed along to the heart.

## The Heart and Circulatory System

As the saying goes, the way to anyone's heart is through the stomach! The Food Qi that rises to the chest (and receives breath from the lungs) nourishes the heart. The heart's energy merges and transforms Food qi with blood, resulting in "Nutritive Qi". Nutritive qi is carried within the blood. The heart directs nutritive qi and blood flow (circulation) through the entire body, moistening and nourishing every organ, tissue, and cell. When this process is unhindered, the heart is relaxed and we experience joy, loving-kindness, and the capacity for happiness. When the heart's energy is contracted or stagnant, we experience feeling disconnected from others, emotional coldness, even hatred.

## The Liver and Gallbladder and Purification System

The liver and gallbladder are important to the digestive process in several ways. When the stomach signals for help because there is too much heat in the small intestine, then the liver and gallbladder contribute cooling salts and bile to restore balance. The liver also purifies and stores the blood. The gallbladder is the assistant. If the liver and gallbladder have too much to purify, they can get congested and stuck. On the emotional level, when the liver gets congested or stagnant, we experience impatience, frustration, bitterness, anger. But when this energy is flowing freely we experience courage, foresight, humor, and flexibility in our thinking.

## The Kidneys and Reproductive System

When Nutritive qi nourishes the kidneys, the hormone system is supported, bones are fortified, urinary function is healthy, and we have physical and mental strength, vitality, willpower, and creativity. If there is not enough qi in the kidney energy system, then we feel afraid in life; we lack willpower and creative drive; and we grow weary of living. Kidney yin and kidney yang are the foundational system of jing energy for the entire body, including the digestive system.

Food qi transforming into Nutritive qi and Defensive qi is primary for every physical function, as well as the emotional, mental, and spiritual dimensions of being human. A combination of systems transforms Nutritive qI into Defensive qi. Warmth from the kidney system, moisture from the stomach, and the integrity of the skin via the lung system together form Defensive qi. (see pg. 110). No life process is separate from our nourishment. Being careful about what we take in — through eating, tasting, seeing, listening, smelling/ breathing, and touching — very much influences our health and well-being — nourishment is mighty. Everything is qi! To embody eating, is to experience the energy connection of all life!

# Friends From Forever II
by David Kailin


steam spirals off congee bowls
rising through the floating motes
struck golden in the morning light


friends from forever rejoin
partaking each other whole
as never parted wonders


attentive as tea unfurls
the wisdom way of water
sip by sip seasons pass by


hot and cold, fans of flavor
full and empty complements
what call, what response is there?


quietudes unite our breath
in spoonfull observations
simply transformed by food

# Acknowledgments

I have been blessed with many excellent mentors along the way of my personal and professional development. The two who have most influenced my knowledge and, more importantly, my understanding of the sophisticated, multidimensional, energetic world of Chinese Medicine are Dr. Richard Tan and Dr. Jeffrey Yuen. Not a day goes by in the clinic when I do not think of these great men and their contribution to this beloved profession for so many practitioners, and for me.

My personal and professional life is supported by my spiritual practice. For over 25 years, my continuous development has been expertly guided by Mary White and Heart Centered Meditation; and my qigong practice by Master Mingtong Gu and Teacher Qifeng Wei for their Zhineng Wisdom Healing Qigong. These three teachers have influenced my life so deeply with their teachings, wisdom, humor, and their being, that I cannot imagine my life without them! Through the loving kindness of my teachers, my life has expanded and grown more happy and healthy. Haola!!

I have felt extremely fortunate in this life to have friends who are such high-quality people, who inspire me, laugh with me, practice with me, help me expand my capacity to grow in my life. I thank you and love you, and trust you know who you are and can smile at this acknowledgment.

To my artist mother, Jean Teare Bright, who created through painting and cooking, and my scientist father, Jack Bright, who appreciated both — thank you! Much love and gratitude for modeling how to enjoy life!

Dr. David Kailin, who, among his many various life achievements, has been a positive force for expanding the profession of Traditional Chinese Medicine into the United States (he holds the Acupuncturist license number 1 for both the state of Washington and Oregon). He has been a teacher, mentor, friend, and also a support to me for writing this book. His poems illustrate the elegant simplicity of his brilliance.

Deep appreciation for my lovely editor, Stephany Wilson. She has kept me focused and inspired, and became a dear friend in the process.

I could not have completed this project without the wise and kind guidance of Nancy Rice, an imaginative and skillful graphic designer, who managed to keep a straight face when I innocently asked her if she thought I could get this whole book done in a few months time! I love her for that alone, and so many other reasons!

To my patients, who are the reason this book was written, I deeply bow in gratitude to you. Your trust in me has given me a livelihood, a sense of purpose, and the ability to practice this medicine that I love. I dearly love you and thank you with my whole heart.

One more acknowledgment, for my family. First, for my husband, Dan. His consistently loving, wise, kind support has made this lifetime a joy for me. And for my children, Jack and Ellen. I thought of them with every recipe, they were my standards for simplicity and flavor; and for cooking with love.

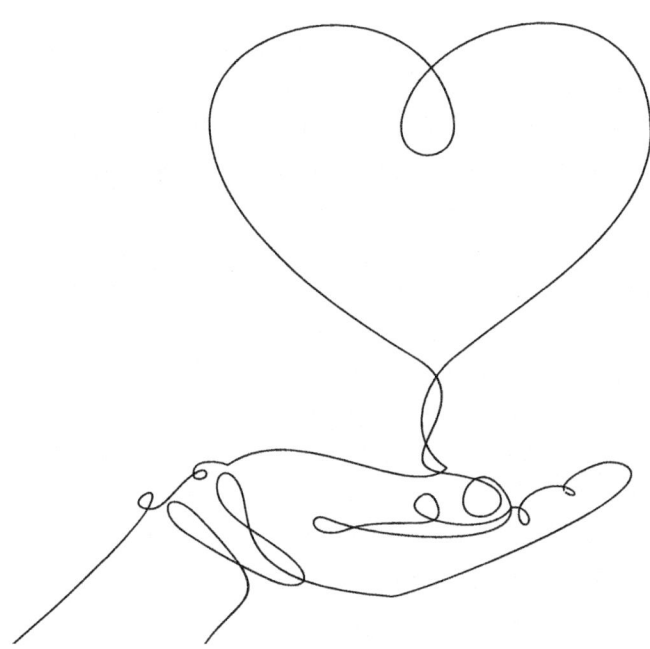

# About the Author

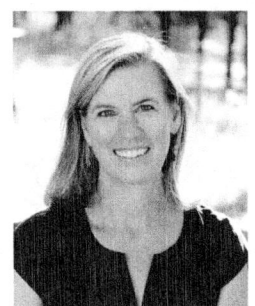

Beth Bright integrates her love of cooking with the wisdom of food properties from Chinese Medicine. Beth has practiced Chinese Medicine for over 2 decades, along with Zhineng Qigong and Meditation. Her combination of interests brings a special quality of expression and understanding to this unique book. Beth lives in Colorado with her husband, children, cat and dog.

Printed in Great Britain
by Amazon

48924364R00071